Immune Intervention

VOLUME 1

New Trends in Vaccines

Immune Intervention

VOLUME 1
New Trends in Vaccines

Edited by

IVAN M. ROITT

Department of Immunology
Middlesex Hospital Medical School
London, England

1984

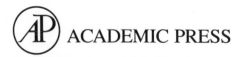 ACADEMIC PRESS

(Harcourt Brace Jovanovich, Publishers)

London   Orlando   San Diego   New York
Toronto   Montreal   Sydney   Tokyo

ACADEMIC PRESS, INC. (LONDON) LTD.
24-28 Oval Road,
London NW1 7DX

United States Edition published by
ACADEMIC PRESS, INC.
Orlando, Florida 32887

LIBRARY OF CONGRESS CATALOG CARD NUMBER: 84-72747

ISBN 0-12-593301-0

PRINTED IN THE UNITED STATES OF AMERICA

84 85 86 87   9 8 7 6 5 4 3 2 1

Contributors

J. W. Almond, *Department of Microbiology, University of Leicester, Leicester, England*

Ruth Arnon, *Department of Chemical Immunology, The Weizmann Institute of Science, Rehovot 76100, Israel*

A. J. Cann, *Department of Microbiology, University of Leicester, Leicester, England*

T. J. R. Harris, *Celltech Ltd., Slough SL1 4DY, England*

F. C. Hay, *Department of Immunology, Middlesex Hospital Medical School, London W1P 9PG, England*

J. H. L. Playfair, *Department of Immunology, Middlesex Hospital Medical School, London W1P 9PG, England*

I. M. Roitt, *Department of Immunology, Middlesex Hospital Medical School, London W1P 9PG, England*

Y. Thanavala, *Department of Immunology, Middlesex Hospital Medical School, London W1P 9PG, England*

Preface

With his customary statesman-like vision, Maurice Landy saw that immunologists are contemplating the application of ideas gleaned from work on experimental models to alter the immunological status of human subjects, whether it be to correct deficiencies or curb excessive responses. He therefore felt that there would be a valuable place for a treatise in which this area was explored and discussed in depth. The appearance of this first volume is a testimony to his efforts.

The contributions in this volume begin with an educational introduction to update the reader and then continue in a rather informal style, probing the subject intensively, thoughtfully and sometimes provocatively, but always reflecting the individuality and independence of the authors.

Vaccination has been immunology's big success story. With the more widespread recognition that the immune system evolved to provide protection against infection, it seemed appropriate to devote this first volume to current problems and trends in the development of new vaccines. The volume contains contributions on the continuing need for vaccines, on attenuation, on the use of gene cloning, on synthetic vaccines, and on idiotype vaccines. I hope it will be read with pleasure and that it will benefit all who have an interest in this subject.

I. M. Roitt

Contents

5 Idiotype Vaccines

F. C. HAY, Y. THANAVALA, AND I. M. ROITT

1

Vaccines: Still Needed

J. H. L. PLAYFAIR

*Department of Immunology,
Middlesex Hospital Medical School,
London, England*

The deviation of Man from the state in which he was originally placed by Nature seems to have proved to him a prolific source of Diseases. From the love of splendour, from the indulgencies of luxury and from his fondness for amusement, he has familiarised himself with a great number of animals, which may not originally have been intended for his associates. The Wolf, disarmed of ferocity, is now pillowed in the lady's lap. The Cat, the little Tyger of our island, whose natural home is the forest, is equally domesticated and caressed. The Cow, the Hog, the Sheep, and the Horse, are all, for a variety of purposes, brought under his care and dominion.

There is a disease to which the Horse, from his state of domestication is frequently subject. . . . it commonly happens that (it) is communicated to the Cows, and from the Cows to the Dairymaids . . . this disease has obtained the name of the Cow Pox . . .

Morbid matter of various kinds, when absorbed into the system, may produce effects in some degree similar but what renders the Cow-pox virus so extremely singular is that the person who has been affected is for ever after secure from the infection of the Small Pox. . . .

Edward Jenner, 1778

On 8 May 1980, the 155 Member states of the World Health Organization represented by their delegates to the Thirty-Third World Health Assembly, unanimously accepted the conclusions of the Global Commission for the Certification of Smallpox eradication—namely that:

1. Smallpox eradication has been achieved throughout the world.
2. There is no evidence that smallpox will return as an endemic disease.

WHO 1980

IMMUNE INTERVENTION

Never in the history of human progress has a better and cheaper method of preventing illness been developed than immunization at its best.

G. Edsall, 1963

Vaccines are no substitute for general improvements in socioeconomic conditions for the control of infectious diseases.

G. Dick, 1978

The phenomenal success of vaccination in ridding the world of smallpox, taming rabies, diphtheria, tetanus, whooping cough, and poliomyelitis and in taking the sting out of meningococcal and pneumococcal disease and tuberculosis should not blind us to the fact that infectious diseases are still the world's principal health problems. There are estimated to be 1800 million people suffering from malaria, 200 million from schistosomiasis, at least 100 million from filariasis, 20 million or more from the various forms of trypanosomiasis, and at least 5 million from leprosy; *all* these diseases are on the increase. George Dick's wise words quoted above notwithstanding, the prospect of the developed countries ever investing the money and effort required to significantly and irreversibly improve the life of their poorer neighbours seems to get less year by year. Therefore, the control of the major tropical diseases by vaccination is still a most desirable and worthwhile aim and has been recognised as such by WHO in the shape of their imaginative Special Programme for Research and Training in Tropical Diseases, which specifically earmarks about one-half of its funds for the development of new vaccines. By a stroke of good fortune, this has happened at a time when two momentous biological advances, gene manipulation, and the production of monoclonal antibodies have opened up undreamed of vistas to the vaccinator. The ways in which these new techniques are being applied to the vaccine problem are the substance of much of this volume; the present brief introduction is intended to show why these and other new ideas are so badly needed by highlighting some of the situations where vaccination is at present not succeeding. These can be roughly classified as follows:

Problems with the vaccine.
    1. Identification of protective antigens.
    2. Cross-reaction and autoimmunity.
    3. Immunogenicity.
    4. Availability.
    5. Safety.
    6. Delivery.
Problems with the immune response.
    7. Immunodeficiency.
    8. Immunosuppression by other diseases.
    9. Immunosuppression by maternal antibody.
   10. Immunopathology.

I. PROTECTIVE ANTIGENS

The identification of antigens was not a pressing problem in the early days of vaccination because either whole intact organisms were used, in an attenuated or inactivated form, or the relevant antigen was obvious, for example, diphtheria and tetanus toxins. The situation is quite different with the majority of protozoal and worm infections, where protection is never more than partial, immunopathology is frequent, and responses are mounted against numerous antigens. Malaria might be cited as typical: the life cycle includes three quite separate forms (sporozoite, asexual blood stage, gametes), each of which may carry up to 20 different antigens; protective immunity can be due to both antibody and a T-dependent nonantibody mechanism, probably involving macrophage activation; immunity does not follow recovery from natural infection except after many years; immune responses are responsible for at least three of the serious complications of the disease (anaemia, glomerulonephritis, and cerebral attacks); and finally, the parasite cannot easily be cultured in bulk (see Section IV). From experiments in laboratory animals, it has been established that vaccination *can* protect against otherwise lethal malaria, but the vaccines are mostly whole parasites or crude extracts, and strong adjuvants are usually needed. This, then, is a case where the identification of antigens that induce protective immunity and not immunopathology is most desirable, and it is no wonder that vaccinators have enthusiastically turned to the monoclonal antibody technique.

A dramatic early success was the purification of a 45,000-MW antigen on the sporozoite of *Plasmodium berghei*, antibody against which protects mice against mosquito-borne infection. Clearly, this constitutes a protective antigen, and one can imagine its bulk synthesis either by chemicals or by gene cloning. With the blood stages, it has long been known that the antibody that blocks entry of the merozoite into the red cell is associated with protection, and passive protection by monoclonal antibodies against *P. yoelii* in mice has now confirmed this. Monoclonal antibodies against human malaria can be tested by the prevention of merozoite invasion *in vitro*, and several antigens of possible value have been isolated. Another approach has been to compare immune and nonimmune sera for their reaction against parasite extracts by crossed electrophoresis in the hope that certain antigens will only be recognized by the immune sera. In this way, at least two antigens, of 65,000 and 90,000 MW have been provisionally identified in *P. knowlesi*-immune monkeys. For a fuller account of these fascinating developments, still in their infancy, the review by Cohen (1982) should be consulted, but it will be obvious that the problem of identifying and purifying antigens corresponding to protective antibody is, in principle, solved; there is no reason to doubt that some kind of vaccine against malaria based on this approach will be available for trial within a few years. This does not mean that malaria will be controlled, because we do not know *how much* of the effective immunity that develops naturally is due to antibody and how much is due to the other mechanisms mentioned earlier, and it cannot be assumed that the antigens that stimulate T cells to activate cytotoxic macrophages or even to become themselves cyto-toxic are the same as those that the antibodies recognise. Indeed, it is often found that purified antigens are relatively feeble immuno-gens for T cells as compared to the living organism. It is noteworthy that the only two successful vaccines so far against intracellular parasites are live attenuated organisms (vaccinia, BCG). Fortu-nately, there are now techniques for cloning T cells, so that in due course it should be possible to test T cells of a single specificity for their ability to protect infected animals. Some success has already been obtained with influenza, and it would be logical to extend this to leprosy, leishmania, South American trypanosomiasis, toxo-plasma, and other intracellular parasites for which no attenuated vaccine at present exists.

A slightly different problem arises with parasites that change their surface antigens either between attacks (e.g., influenza) or during the infection itself (e.g., African trypanosomes). Experi-ments with cloned trypanosomes in mice suggest that a killed vaccine can protect against the homologous variant, yet all attempts to use mixtures of variants as vaccines in cattle have been unsuc-cessful. Depressingly, the estimate of the number of variant genes available to the trypanosome has risen from about 50 to nearer 1000, whereas with influenza there is suspected to be a reservoir of animal viruses with which the human virus exchanges genetic material. In such cases, the concept of protective antigens rather loses its meaning, but several workers are searching optimistically for some shred of constancy against which to vaccinate; here again the monoclonal antibody technique shows the way, with its ability to pick out and amplify one specificity from thousands.

II. CROSS-REACTING ANTIGENS AND AUTOIMMUNITY

Several parasitic organisms share antigens with their host, which is then placed in the dilemma of whether to suppress its response or to respond and destroy itself. One example of the latter risk is the damage to heart and neural tissue in Chagas' disease due to cross-reaction between these organs and *Trypanosoma cruzi*. Vac-cination with the whole parasite might further stimulate the autoim-munity without necessarily eliminating the infection, which would be a very poor bargain. Encouragingly, a glycoprotein has been purified that will protect mice against *T. cruzi* but that does not cross-react with any host antigen, and once again monoclonal antibodies offer a quick and easy way of checking for this in other cases.

It is not only with microorganisms that the problem of cross-reaction arises. One approach to fertility control might be to immunise women against chorionic gonadotrophin (hCG), whose presence is vital to maintain pregnancy. Unfortunately, this molecule shares its alpha chain with several other hormones, including thyroid stimulating hormone (TSH), and even its beta chain has extensive homology with that of luteinizing hormone (LH), only 35 out of 145 amino acids being exclusive to hCG. A peptide of about 35 amino acids should therefore be a safe vaccine, though of course such small molecules need help from carriers and adjuvants (see Section III).

The ultimate in antigen sharing is the tumour cell, which in most cases probably does not display any antigens not found on the corresponding normal tissue, though sometimes the sharing is only with a small number of precursors (e.g., the acute lymphoid leukemia antigen found on stem cells). One exception is the malignant B lymphocyte, whose Ig idiotype constitutes a true "tumour-specific antigen," and one remarkable example of treatment by anti-idiotype serum has been reported (Miller *et al.*, 1982).

III. IMMUNOGENICITY

The 35-amino acid peptide mentioned above is an extreme case, but it is a general rule that small molecules on their own are far less antigenic than whole organisms. Presumably, this is largely due to the carrier effect of other microbial antigens, and one solution is to couple the peptide to a molecule of proven immunogenicity, such as tetanus toxoid or Keyhole Limpet haemocyanin. The latter has been used with conspicuous success in guinea pigs as a carrier for a 20-amino acid synthetic peptide from the foot-and-mouth disease virus (Bittle *et al.*, 1982). The same approach may be called for even with quite large molecules that fail to stimulate T helper cells, such as the new pneumococcal and meningococcal polysaccharide vaccines, which display rather variable immunogenicity and induce little or no memory. It would be worth some trouble to establish a panel of safe and effective carrier molecules for human use. The same is true for adjuvants, because despite extensive work, the only ones in routine use are still aluminium hydroxide (with toxoids) and *Bordetella pertussis*, which probably improves the response to diphtheria and tetanus in the triple vaccine. Great hopes are placed on the various water-soluble derivatives of the tubercle bacillus, such as muramyl dipeptide, both as adjuvants and as direct macrophage activators, but it is too early to say how good they really are. In the monkey malaria model referred to earlier, nothing has so far been able to consistently replace Freund's complete adjuvant.

IV. AVAILABILITY

The reluctance of many parasites to grow *in vitro* or in suitable animals constitutes a severe stumbling block to antigen preparation. Patient observation can occasionally overcome this—who would have guessed that the nine-banded armadillo would become a laboratory animal because of its ability to grow vast numbers of leprosy bacilli? But with most worms, for example, whose complex life cycle involving insect or snail vectors cannot be bypassed in the laboratory as can the insect vectors of protozoa, the production of large amounts of antigen is a formidable undertaking. Even the culture of *P. falciparum* malaria, which is now being carried out in hundreds of laboratories around the world, is proving very difficult to scale up to the sort of yields required by commerce. Of course, this may not matter once protective antigens have been identified, but this in turn is only possible where reasonable experimental models of immunity exist, as they do for malaria. A good example of a parasite, where no animal model remotely resembles the human disease, is *Onchocerca volvulus*, the dreaded cause of River Blindness, though experiments are struggling ahead, *faute de mieux*, in cattle.

V. SAFETY

It has been said that if aspirin were discovered tomorrow it would never be licensed for sale, and one is often struck, at international meetings, by the contrast between the horror of theoretically possible complications of vaccination in the laboratories where they are produced and the more philosophical attitude of those in the affected countries who would administer them. We certainly cannot afford disasters such as bedevilled diphtheria toxin–antitoxin mixtures in the 1920s, the early "inactivated" polio vaccines, yellow fever vaccine in 1942 (contaminated with hepatitis virus), or BCG in the Lubeck tragedy of 1930 (an administrative mix-up). Likewise nobody would consider using Freund's complete adjuvant. But the controversy over pertussis vaccine (Stewart, 1977; Kaplan *et al.*, 1979) shows that a vaccine can hold its own despite undisputed side effects.

VI. DELIVERY

In a classic study, McBean *et al.* (1976) investigated over 1000 children in Cameroon who were vaccinated against measles. Of these, 44% already had antibody whereas 25% failed to respond, indicating that the vaccine had lost effectiveness somewhere between the factory (in the United States) and the clinic. In addition, 14% of vaccine doses were not used. Thus, only about one dose in six achieved its purpose. Measles vaccine is particularly susceptible to refrigeration breakdown, but the moral is plain: if delivery fails, money spent on research and manufacture is wasted.

VII. IMMUNODEFICIENCY

The use of live attenuated vaccines in immunodeficient children has introduced clinicians to some gruesome new diseases whose names speak for themselves: vaccinia gangrenosa, giant cell pneumonia of measles, miliary BCGosis. The current practice of giving BCG at birth in tropical countries means that inevitably the rare child with congenital T-cell deficiency will be put at risk, but of course it is very unlikely that such children would survive for long in any case. Infinitely more common is the immunodeficiency of malnutrition, though the link between nutritional status and response to vaccination is not as simple as might be anticipated. Children who are merely underweight seem to respond fairly

normally to most vaccines, but where protein deficiency predomi-
nates, as in Kwashiokor and Marasmus, antibody responses are
diminished and protection is likely to be inadequate following most
bacterial and viral vaccines. The very real problem of whether to
protect undernourished children against endemic measles by active
or passive immunization is discussed in the excellent chapter on
Immunization in Greenwood and Whittle (1981). There is also a
tendency to inadequate delayed-type hypersensitivity reactions in
patients who are deficient in protein, iron, or zinc, which can cause
confusion when skin testing for tuberculosis, etc., though it does not
follow that because the skin test remains negative no protection has
been induced, and indeed to establish the point would take many
years, which might better be spent trying to correct the deficiencies.

VIII. IMMUNOSUPPRESSION

People in tropical countries rarely suffer from a single disease,
and many diseases strikingly affect immunity to other diseases. The
best-known examples are malaria, trypanosomiasis, and measles,
all of which induce strong nonspecific immunosuppression, but
milder degrees have been reported in almost every known infectious disease. Mechanisms vary. With the above-mentioned protozoa, suppression of both antibody and T-cell responses is mainly
due to the products of highly activated macrophages, including
prostaglandins, but in measles part of the defect is probably due to
actual infection of lymphocytes by the virus. But whatever the
mechanism, the effects can be critical for the vaccinator; one strik-
ing instance is the poor antibody responses to Salmonella and
Meningococcal vaccines in children with malaria (Williamson and
Greenwood, 1978). Suppression of immunity to the Epstein-Barr
virus by malaria may also account for the virtual restriction of
Burkitt's lymphoma to the malaria belt, another very good reason
for trying to eliminate malaria!

The great variability of protection by BCG against tuberculosis
in different parts of the world is also attributed by some workers to
a subtle form of interference induced by other mycobacteria in the
environment. For example in Uganda, where BCG is highly effective, *Mycobacterium chromogenicum* and *M. vaccae* are plentiful,

whereas in Burma and South India, where a recent large BCG trial was a complete failure, *M. scrofulaceum* and *M. kansasii* abound. The argument (Stanford *et al.*, 1981) is that these other organisms, which tend to induce "Listeria type" (protective) and "Koch type" (necrotic) responses, respectively, also predispose to the corresponding type of response to TB. The same authors have suggested that mycobacterial contamination of drinking water might also lead to specific immunosuppression. These considerations might have great significance for vaccination against leprosy because BCG is at present the only vaccine with any effect against this disease.

IX. MATERNAL ANTIBODY

Interference by passively acquired maternal antibody with the development of active immunity by the newborn is a well established phenomenon that needs to be taken into account in planning the timing of first vaccination. It is for this reason that measles vaccination is usually not given before 1 year of age. However in many tropical countries measles is endemic, so that to immunise children effectively requires almost split-second timing. Another disease where this problem will certainly arise is malaria. Harte *et al.* (1982, 1983) have shown that titres of maternal IgG, such as are commonly found in Africans, will completely prevent protection by vaccination in a mouse model. In analysing the mechanism of this, they found it to be partly due to a direct effect of antibody on the handling of the vaccine after injection and partly due to the induction of specific suppressor T cells, which act to inhibit the malaria-specific helper T cells (Harte *et al.*, 1983). In both mouse and man, the only class of maternal immunoglobulin to enter the neonatal circulation is IgG, and this appears to be an extremely efficient inducer of suppressor T cells, probably as part of its ordinary regulatory role. It was also found that specific IgM could to some extent overcome this, and these authors suggested that IgM (monoclonal of course!) might be given with the vaccine instead of waiting until the maternal IgG had disappeared. The possibilities of IgM and other adjuvants in advancing the potential age of vaccination constitute an urgent subject for research in relation to almost every tropical infection.

X. IMMUNOPATHOLOGY

One of the nightmares of the vaccinator exploring unknown territory is that his efforts will make the patient worse, especially with diseases that people have come to accept as part of normal life. One can imagine the impact in Britain or the United States of a vaccine against the common cold that gave its victims asthma! Yet this is no worse than some of the possible consequences of immunising against many parasites without completely eliminating them. For instance a vaccine against *T. cruzi* might exacerbate autoimmune myocarditis (see Section II); a schistosome vaccine that contained egg antigen might hasten the onset of the liver cirrhosis, which is the only serious manifestation of this disease; filarial vaccines might make elephantiasis or choroidoretinitis even more crippling and horrible than they already are. Less certain, but always to be borne in mind, is the possibility that enhanced antibody responses will lead to enhanced levels of immune complexes and kidney disease. In short, wherever there is immunopathology in the disease there will have to be purified antigens in the vaccine.

I hope this brief review has illustrated the wide range of diseases still awaiting the vaccinator and some of the difficulties in store for him; it also indicates the resurgence of interest in research in laboratories around the world. I very much doubt whether the next big breakthrough will have to wait, as did Pasteur's anthrax vaccine after Jenner's vaccinia, nearly 100 years!

REFERENCES

Bittle J. L., Houghten, R. A., Alexander, H., Shinnick, T. M., Sutcliffe, J. G., Lerner, A., Rowlands, D. J. and Brown, F. (1982). *Nature (London)* **298,** 30–33.

Cohen, S. (1982). *Br. Med. Bull.* **38,** 161–165.

Greenwood, B. M. and Whittle, H. C. (1981). "Immunology of Medicine in the Tropics." Edward Arnold, London.

Harte, P. G. and Playfair, J. H. L. (1983). *Clin. Exp. Immunol.* **51,** 157–164.

Harte, P. G., De Souza, J. B. and Playfair, J. H. L. (1982). *Clin. Exp. Immunol.* **49,** 509–516.

Harte, P. G., Cooke, A. and Playfair, J. H. L. (1983). *Nature (London)* **302,** 256–258.

Kaplan, J. P., Schoenbaum, S. C., Weinstein, M. C. and Fraser, D. W. (1979). *New Engl. J. Med.* **301,** 906–911.

McBean, A. M., Foster, S. O., Herrman, K. L. and Gateef, C. (1976). *Trans. Roy. Soc. Trop. Med. Hyg.* **70,** 206–212.
Miller, R. A., Maloney, D. G., Warnke, R. and Levy, R. (1982). *New Engl. J. Med.* **306,** 517–522.
Stanford, J. L., Shield, M. J. and Rook, G. A. W. (1981). *Tubercle* **62,** 55–62.
Stewart, G. T. (1977). *Lancet* **i,** 234–237.
Williamson, W. A. and Greenwood, B. M. (1978). *Lancet* **i,** 1328–1329.

2

Attenuation

J. W. ALMOND AND A. J. CANN

Department of Microbiology,
University of Leicester,
Leicester, England

I. INTRODUCTION

A. Definitions

Attenuation can be defined as the process of weakening the characteristic force of an entity. In the context of microbiology, attenuation refers to a reduction in the capacity of an organism to cause disease, or a diminution of its characteristic pathogenicity. The attenuation of pathogenic microorganisms as a basis for vaccine design and development is a long-established alternative to the use of noninfectious antigenic mass in the form of killed, split, subunit, or synthetic preparations. The extent to which a microorganism can be attenuated is limited by the practical constraints of immunoprophylaxis. Obviously, its capacity to cause disease must be substan-

IMMUNE INTERVENTION
Copyright © 1984 by Academic Press, London
All rights of reproduction in any form reserved
ISBN 0-12-593301-0

tially diminished, but a microorganism so radically attenuated that it is no longer capable of infecting its natural host would be useless for vaccine purposes. Microorganisms ideally attenuated for vaccine use can be defined as those possessing the following properties. First, the organism must be capable of establishing an infection in the desired host following artificial administration. This should mimic the natural infection as closely as possible in stimulating all facets of the immune response (most notably immunological memory). Second, the organism should have lost the capacity to produce anything but the mildest of disease symptoms and, in addition, should be free of any undesirable secondary characteristics that might limit its use as a live vaccine, such as the ability to cause rare malignancies or to establish a persistent or latent infection. Also, ideally, an attenuated organism should be free from teratogenic or abortogenic effects. Third, the attenuated microorganism's propensity for spread to contacts and dissemination throughout a population should be as low as possible. Finally, the organism should be very stable genetically and thereby be virtually incapable of reverting to a virulent form.

Thus, an ideal live-attentuated vaccine would cause a mild or inapparent infection of the vaccinee only, would stimulate, from a single inoculation, a long-lasting immune response protective against the wild-type disease, and would be totally free of any undesirable side effects for the individual recipient and for the population as a whole.

B. The Case for Live-Attenuated Vaccines

In considering strategies for the development of vaccines, the relative merits of live-attenuated versus killed preparations of microorganisms are being continually debated (e.g., Salk and Salk, 1978). The most notable arguments in this debate are those concerned with immunogenicity or efficacy of the material, safety, ease of production, distribution, administration, stability, and cost. Such discussions are of course entirely pertinent for each individual microorganism, but ought not to lead to policy decisions to cover vaccines as a whole. Each infectious disease is caused by a unique and characteristic microorganism, which stimulates its own range and balance of nonspecific and specific cellular and humoral immune responses. Depending on the nature of these responses and their relative roles in pathogenesis, recovery, and subsequent protection from the disease, a particular type of vaccine against a given disease may be either appropriate or useless. For example, early, killed measles vaccine was considered promising by the criterion that it induced good serum neutralizing antibody and probably also a cell-mediated response (Fulginiti and Arthur, 1969; Harris *et al.*, 1969). However, although recipients appeared to be protected for 3 to 5 years postvaccination, later they lost their resistance and, upon infection, developed a more severe form of the disease known as atypical measles (Cherry *et al.*, 1972). It has been suggested that residual immunity, which was mainly cellular (Isacson and Stone, 1971), together with a rapidly developing secondary serum-antibody response, probably gave rise to this modified immunopathology (Chanock and Richman, 1975). An alternative explanation is provided by the finding that in killed vaccine preparations, the immunogenicity of one of the surface glycoproteins (the fusion protein) was destroyed, and therefore only partial immunity was induced (Norrby, 1975; Norrby *et al.*, 1975; Norrby and Lagercrantz, 1976). Subsequently, live-attenuated vaccines have been highly successful in reducing the incidence of measles, particularly in the United States and the U.S.S.R. (Witte and Axnick, 1975; Burgastow *et al.*, 1973).

A comparable observation has been made with respiratory syncytial virus (RSV). In spite of receiving inactivated material that induced high levels of neutralising antibody and a vigorous cell-mediated immune response, vaccinees suffered severe RSV lower respiratory tract disease more often than did unvaccinated cohorts (Kim *et al.*, 1969; Kapikian *et al.*, 1969). Here again, an unbalanced immunological response was the most probable explanation of this phenomenon. An inadequate stimulation of localised immunity would account for the vaccinees being unprotected against wild-type infection, whereas the vigorous systemic immune response probably provided the basis for immunopathological damage (Chanock, 1976). It remains to be seen whether a live-attenuated respiratory syncytial virus will make a more effective vaccine (Wright *et al.*, 1970), but since individuals who recover from the natural infection are not reinfected, it may be assumed that some component of the immune response not stimulated by the killed vaccine (probably secretary IgA) must confer protection.

These examples illustrate the need, in certain circumstances, to provide a complete and balanced immune response in order to ensure adequate defence against disease. On the other hand, the use of toxoids as vaccines provides an example in which the use of inactivated material is highly effective. Infection by an attenuated organism is thought to stimulate a very similar array of immune responses to the natural infection, including cell-mediated and secretory antibody responses that may not normally be induced by injection of killed antigen.

The quality of the immune response to live-attenuated-versus-killed vaccines is therefore very important. In general, systemic immunity probably provides effective protection against microorganisms during the course of infection with which there is a systemic spread of the whole organism or some component of it (e.g., yellow fever, polio, tetanus, diphtheria). However, the importance of stimulating local immunity to provide protection at the site of entry (e.g., alimentary or respiratory tracts) against organisms that undergo such spread or, indeed, to protect against infections that remain predominantly localised (e.g., rhinoviruses, rotaviruses, *Escherichia coli*) should not be overlooked, especially because protection against infection, rather than mere protection against the disease, may be of greater benefit to the population as a whole.

Antigenic mass is another factor in light of which live-attenuated vaccines seem particularly attractive. For killed vaccines, a measured amount of antigen, either microgram quantities of a purified antigen or milligram quantities of a killed whole organism, are required to stimulate a protective antibody response. By contrast, the dose of live-attentuated vaccine required is usually measured in units of infectious dose (ID_{50}) and in terms of antigen amount may be orders of magnitude smaller than its killed counterpart. From the point of view of vaccine production procedures, cost, and administration, this difference in dose size is highly significant, especially since for killed vaccines two or three doses are often required to give the primary and secondary responses that normally preceed long-lasting immunity. With live-attenuated vaccines, a single dose is usually sufficient because primary and secondary responses are merged together during amplification of the administered dose.

The use of live-attenuated vaccines does have certain disadvantages however. Propagating live microorganisms and distributing them throughout the environment can never be totally free of hazard. For example, genetic stability of vaccines is of major concern. Attenuated microorganisms must remain attenuated upon replication within the vaccinee. Even a very low level of reversion, such as, for instance, that which is sufficient to give one case of disease from 1×10^5 administered doses, may be regarded as unacceptably high if that case forms a focal point of an outbreak of disease. Such risks should not, in principle, be encountered with killed vaccines.

Vaccination against poliomyelitis probably provides the best available assessment of the relative merits of live versus inactivated vaccines (Salk and Salk, 1978; World Health Organization, 1982). Problems associated with the use of OPV have included contamination with other viruses (Sweet and Hilleman, 1960), interference from other gut infections, and the instability during transit to outlying areas. These last two problems are particularly severe in many underdeveloped countries (Sabin, 1956; Oduntan *et al.*, 1978; Bazin, 1980). Perhaps the major cause for concern, however, is vaccine-associated disease. Available evidence suggests that live polio vaccines cause approximately one case of paralysis per 6.7×10^6 administered doses (World Health Organization, 1982). Viruses isolated (usually serotype 3) from these rare cases can be designated "vaccine-like" on biochemical and serological criteria (Minor, 1980, 1982; Kew *et al.*, 1980). In countries using killed vaccine exclusively, such viruses are not encountered.

For many live-attenuated vaccines for use in humans, medical circumstances exist under which their use is contraindicated. Thus in individuals with almost any disorder of the immune system, in individuals immunosupressed by other means, in pregnant women, and in geriatrics, the use of live-vaccines such as polio, rubella, measles, and influenza would be ill-advised. Similarly, smallpox vaccine was not recommended for individuals suffering from eczema. During mass vaccination programmes such high-risk groups are potentially at risk from the live vaccines administered to close contacts. In practice, this risk is minimized by using vaccines of as low transmissability as possible, although there is good evidence of incidents of disease after contact with vaccinees (World Health Organization, 1982). Another attraction of vaccines of low transmissability is that they will be limited in their opportunity to interact genetically with wild-type related organisms. Fears that novel recombinants of unpredictable pathogenicity may result from such interactions have been voiced in the case of the influenza viruses (Scholtissek, 1978).

The case for live-attenuated versus killed vaccine must therefore be debated for each individual disease, taking account of all the factors relating to the microorganism and its pathogenesis and of the response of the host to it.

II. HISTORICAL AND GENERAL PRINCIPLES

A. Early Examples

To trace the history of attenuation of microorganisms for vaccine development is to trace the history of vaccination itself. Probably the earliest form of vaccination, performed by the Chinese over a 1000 years ago, was the practice of variolation; the inoculation of susceptible nonimmune individuals with the pustular exudate from patients suffering from smallpox (see Langer, 1976; Baxby, 1981). Whilst naturally occurring rather than intentionally attenuated strains were used for this purpose, the general procedure was to obtain infectious material from a particularly mild case of smallpox and to pass this material from one individual to the next. It is likely that, in the interest of safety, exudate from the few individuals who developed the generalised disease as a result of variolation would have been avoided. The procedure was of course not without risk, not only to the individual recipients involved but also to the community at large, and there is some evidence of its association with the foci of small outbreaks of smallpox. It is interesting to note that there were improvements in the success of variolation as the practice became widespread in Britain, Europe, and the United States during the eighteenth century. Of the patients inoculated by Zabdiel Boyston at Boston in 1721, approximately 1 in 50 died. Half a century later, Robert and Daniel Sutton reported that they had inoculated 2514 individuals in England during the 1760s without a single fatality. It is conceivable that, during the passage from one individual to the next, variants that had become mildly attenuated *in vivo* were selected. However, such improvements in the success rate may have also been due to improvements in the methods of inoculating individuals. The practice of variolation was abandoned in the early nineteenth century with the advent of Jenner and his discovery that nature provides its own comparatively safe live vaccine against smallpox in the form of the naturally attenuated cowpox and vaccinia viruses.

The earliest observations that microorganisms could be purposefully attenuated in their capacity to cause disease were made by Pasteur in the 1870s and 1880s. Although some of Pasteur's "attenuations" were probably made by killing the offending pathogen while retaining its antigenicity, undoubtedly Pasteur made the first real progress towards the production of live-attenuated microorganisms for use as vaccines. He found that when a strain of *Bacillus anthracis* was grown in broth culture at 42–43°C, it not only lost its capacity to produce spores, but after 2 to 3 months became nonpathogenic for cattle and sheep. In 1881 Pasteur demonstrated that animals inoculated with this culture could be protected from the usually fatal anthrax that followed injection with a virulent strain. A few years later, Pasteur illustrated a procedure that was subsequently of great benefit in attenuation, especially of viruses, that of alternative host adaption. Although his final vaccine against rabies was air-dried and therefore probably killed material, the virus had been adapted to grow rapidly in rabbit brain (causing death of the animal within 7 days). Pasteur, in collaboration with Chamberland and Roux, had also noticed that if rabies was passed from dog to monkey and then from monkey to monkey, its virulence for dog, rabbit, or guinea pig fell with each passage. Furthermore, rabies attenuated in this way could be used to make dogs refractory to virulent strains (see Steele, 1975). These experiments set the stage for the development of attenuated microorganisms for vaccine purposes.

Notable early advances included the development of a live-attenuated vaccine against tuberculosis: the BCG (Bacille Calmet-Guerin) in 1921. This was achieved by prolonged cultivation of a virulent bovine strain of the tubercle bacilli on glycerol–potato medium to which bile had been added, an ingredient that had been observed earlier to induce a change in colony morphology. After 231 subcultures over a period of 13 years, the resulting bacteria could be injected into animals and man without causing anything more than a retrogressive lesion, while stimulating some degree of immunity towards *Mycobacterium tuberculosis*.

The most notable early success against a virus disease of humans was made by Theiler with the yellow fever virus. The 17-D vaccine, highly successful and still in use today, was developed by multiple passage of wild-type yellow fever virus initially in mouse embryo tissue culture, then in chick embryo tissue culture, and finally in tissue culture prepared from chick embryos from which the brains and spinal cords had been removed. This procedure was deemed to have reduced the viscerotropic and neurotropic properties of the virus. The resulting strain failed to kill monkeys and required an increased incubation period to cause encephalitis in mice (Theiler and Smith 1937). Later, studies on pathogenesis in rhesus monkeys showed that the attenuated strain multiplied to a lower titre than wild-type in lymphoid tissue and bone marrow and unusually, failed to infect the vital target site of virulent yellow fever virus—the liver.

B. General Principles

The past few decades have seen the attenuation of many pathogenic microorganisms for development of medical and veterinary vaccines. Included are representatives of most of the major families of viruses, i.e., picornaviridae, calciviridae, orthomyxoviridae, paramyxoviridae, reoviridae, parvoviridae, adenoviridae, and herpesviridae; a smaller number of bacteria, e.g., *Bacillus anthracis, Bordetella bronchoseptica, Brucella abortis, Erysipelothrix insidiosa, Salmonella* sp., *Mycobacteria* sp., plus an occasional example of mycoplasma, e.g., *Mycoplasma mycoides*. Rather than attempt to give comprehensive documentation on the attenuation of all of these microorganisms, the remainder of this article will primarily concentrate on those that are used as vaccines in humans. Because, with only the one exception already discussed (BCG), these are viruses, relatively little discussion will be devoted to the attenuation of bacteria. A comprehensive list of live-attenuated veterinary vaccines and a discussion of the attenuation of bacteria can be found in Buxton and Frazer (1978).

The examples described in the remainder of this article have been attenuated by variations on, or combinations of, the general methods given below. These methods were developed mainly in the 1950s and 1960s during the surge of progress in virology that accompanied the application of tissue culture techniques. This period saw the development of most of the live-attenuated vaccines in current medical use. Attenuation was, and to some extent remains, a rather empirical phenomenon. However, although initial attempts to achieve it were based largely on trial and error, there was a common rationale, i.e., to produce variants that grow optimally under conditions slightly different to those found in the natural host cell. It was found that many such variants became less suited for growth in their original host and, therefore, although able to stimulate immunity, were unable to replicate efficiently enough to cause disease. There is no doubt that the realization that many pathogenic microorganisms could be attenuated, together with the availability of attenuated strains for studies *in vitro,* contributed significantly to the conception of virus-induced disease. Lwoff (1959, 1969) and Sabin (1961) placed great emphasis on the ability of virulent microorganisms to withstand the changes in local pH and body temperature that occurred during an inflammatory response. Evidence of a correlation between the inability to replicate at low pH and at 39 to 40°C *in vitro* and reduced virulence *in vivo* was obtained for a number of viruses (Melnick *et al.,* 1958; Vogt *et al.,* 1957; Kilham, 1959; Lwoff, 1959; Rohitayodhin and Hammon, 1962; Hozinski *et al.,* 1966). Thus, purposeful modification of the pH optimum for growth, or more frequently, the temperature optimum for growth *in vitro* became general methods to accompany the already established procedure of alternative host adaption.

1. Adaption to a Foreign Host or Tissue. Although for some pathogens, such as those that naturally possess a broad host range, it is possible to produce characteristic clinical symptoms immediately upon inoculation into a laboratory animal (e.g., cowpox on rabbit skin or on the chorioallantois of hen's eggs), for most microorganisms it is necessary first to adapt them to the new host by repeated passage. It was observed very early on that a frequent consequence of such adaptation was a coincidental attenuation of the microorganisms for its original host. Thus alternative host adaption became one of the first widely used methods for attenuating microorganisms (Fenner and Cairns, 1959).

Early examples were based on passage in a foreign host *in vivo,* but the success rates of such procedures were generally poor, probably because of encounters with nonspecific and specific immune defence mechanisms during the period of very slow growth of the organism in early passage. Propagation *in vitro* has proved much more successful, and now almost all currently used live-attenuated vaccines have a history of passage in laboratory culture.

The conditions used for attenuating viruses by this method have varied enormously. Success seems to depend on the characteristics of the virus under study, the alternative host cell culture system used, and the number and conditions of passage. Schemes have been developed largely as a result of trial and error, and it is unclear why in some cases attenuation is achieved rapidly and predictably, whereas in other cases protracted passage in a number of different hosts and tissue types may be required. The only rules currently adhered to, especially for the development of human vaccines, are that, in the interests of safety, viruses should at no stage be passaged in permanent aneuploid cell lines, in cells derived from tumour tissue, or in cells known to be persistently infected by another virus or by mycoplasma. Primary cells should be prepared from animals that are specified pathogen-free (see World Health Organization, 1981).

The simplest procedure to achieve attenuation of a virus involves a mere manipulation of its tissue tropism by repeated passage in cells of the original host derived from organs not involved in major pathology. For example, repeated passage of Marek's disease virus, which causes a lymphoproliferative disease of chickens, in primary chicken kidney cells in culture, resulted in a loss of oncogenicity after about 30 passages. Virus obtained after passage number 60 was found to be suitably attenuated for vaccine use (Churchill *et al.,* 1969a,b). This procedure, for reasons not understood, obviously selected for apathogenic mutants that were able to outgrow the parent virus in the culture system used. Antigenic differences observed between the attenuated variant and its virulent parent had little consequence to the stimulation of immunity, and the strain proved effective as a vaccine for a number of years before being replaced by a naturally occurring apathogenic virus, the herpes virus of turkeys (Purchase, 1976).

A further example in which attenuation can be achieved rapidly and confidently is with mumps virus. Following observations by Enders *et al.* (1949), the presently used live vaccine, the Jeryl Lynn strain, developed at Merck, Sharpe and Dohme laboratories, was found to be sufficiently attenuated for vaccine use after 17 passages in the amniotic cavity or chick embryo fibroblasts from leukosis-free eggs (Bunyak and Hilleman, 1966). In this case again, the degree of attenuation seems to be directly proportional to the number of passages, and continued propagation leads to the generation of over-attenuated variants incapable of producing an adequate immune response in humans.

The arbitrary nature of the experimental schemes that can be used to produce attenuated strains is illustrated by the case of rubella virus. Following the first successful propagation of this virus in cell culture in 1962 (Weller and Neva, 1962) and the enormous stimulus provided by the devastating rubella epidemic in the United States in 1963–1964, several groups almost simultaneously began to develop live-attenuated vaccines. Three different strains are currently in use as vaccines (see Huygelen, 1978). The HPV-77 strain was attenuated by 77 passages in primary green monkey kidney cells (Parkman *et al.*, 1966). Because of fears concerning the possible contamination of these cells with simian viruses and occasional reactogenicity during trials in humans, this strain was passaged further in duck embryo fibroblasts (Bunyak *et al.*, 1968). The resulting virus, designated HPV-77/DE5, has been widely used. A second rubella vaccine, the Cendehill strain, was obtained by making 51 passages of the virus in primary rabbit kidney cells (Huygelen and Peetermans, 1967). The third strain, RA 27/3, was attenuated by 25 passages in the WI-38 strain of human diploid cells (Plotkin *et al.*, 1967). Each of these viruses provides a vaccine that is immunogenic, sufficiently attenuated, and unable to spread to contacts of recipients. It is clear then that attenuation of a single virus can be achieved by several experimental procedures.

Details of the passage histories that have led to the attenuation of many viruses are available, e.g., Venezuelan equine encephalitis virus (Koprowski and Leuneffe, 1946), measles virus (Enders *et al.,* 1960), cytomegalovirus (Elek and Stern, 1974), varicella virus (Takahashi *et al.,* 1974), and hepatitis A virus (Provost *et al.,* 1982), but of themselves, they provide little illustration of how, why, or when attenuation occurs. It is unclear why such procedures can be applied with apparent ease to some viruses and yet are consistently less than successful even with closely related viruses, e.g., polio as compared with foot-and-mouth disease virus. Obviously a series of mutations occur during protracted passage in culture. The precise molecular effects of these mutations and the reasons why they occur during *in vitro* passage are not yet understood.

2. *Adaption to Growth at Suboptimal Temperature.* Although one of Pasteur's original successes, the attenuation of *Bacillus anthracis,* was achieved by passage at elevated temperature, evidence that opposite effects may be obtained with viruses (Armstrong, 1929; Armstrong and Lillie, 1929) led to attempts to bring about attenuation by adaptation to growth at temperatures lower than that of the body of the natural host (Dubes and Chapin, 1956). It was observed that strains of all three serotypes of poliovirus could be adapted to growth at 23°C in monkey kidney cell cultures and that the resulting "cold-adapted strains" had reduced neurovirulence for monkeys when injected intraspinally (Dubes and Wenner, 1957). For these and other cold-adapted viruses (Rohitayodhin and Hammon, 1962), it also was noticed that the strains frequently lost their ability to replicate at temperatures around 39 to 40°C. According to Lwoff (1959, 1969), this temperature sensitivity represents a major factor contributing to reduced pathogenicity, and accordingly a simple test *in vitro,* the replicative capacity test (rct/40°C), became a widely used genetic marker of reduced virulence (see Hozinski *et al.,* 1966).

Procedures used to cold-adapt viruses in culture varied in detail for each cell–virus system under study, but broadly followed the scheme of Dubes and Wenner (1957). Stepwise reduction in temperature of incubation by 2 to 3°C, after heavy inoculation of the culture, interspersed by 1 to 10 passages at that temperature, usually proved sucessful. At various stages, plaque purification and/ or passage at terminal end-point dilution was used to select for adapted variants. A sudden sharp drop in temperature was generally found to be unsuccessful (e.g., Maassab, 1967), suggesting that cold adaptation resulted from an accumulation of several mutations. Final selection temperatures varied from 23°C for polio viruses (Dubes and Wenner, 1957), 25°C for influenza viruses (Maassab, 1967), and 33°C for rubella virus (Plotkin *et al.*, 1967). Because of the belief that it is the temperature-sensitive character of cold-adapted strains that is primarily responsible for their reduced virulence, some workers have taken the shortcut of screening directly for either spontaneously occurring or mutagen-induced, temperature-sensitive mutants from a wild-type virus population (Burge and Pfefferkorn, 1966; Cooper, 1964; Fried, 1965). Temperature-sensitive mutants of many viruses have been isolated and administered to animals; these include polioviruses (Ghendon *et al.*, 1973), influenza viruses (Mackenzie, 1970; Mills *et al.*, 1969; Markushin and Ghendon, 1973), reovirus (Fields, 1972), parainfluenza viruses (Potash *et al.*, 1970; Zygraich *et al.*, 1972), respiratory syncytial virus (Wright *et al.*, 1970), herpes simplex virus (Zygraich and Huygelen, 1973), vesicular stomatitis virus (Wagner, 1974), and rabies virus (Selimov and Nikitina, 1970). As discussed in greater detail for influenza viruses in the next section, almost all of these mutants show a reduction in pathogenicity. However, because they arise mainly through single point mutations, genetic instability can present a serious problem to the use of these strains as vaccines.

III. EXAMPLES OF CURRENT RESEARCH

As will be discussed in Section IV, research on attenuation is inextricably linked to research on microbial pathogenicity. It is not the purpose of this review to deal with the latter subject and several excellent articles can be found elsewhere (e.g., Rott, 1979; Smith *et al.*, 1980; Fields and Green, 1982). Rather than attempt to cover present research on the attenuation of all microorganisms, two examples have been chosen for detailed consideration. The first example, that of the influenza A viruses, is beset by the problem of antigenic variation, probably the major reason why, in spite of much effort over the past two decades, a live-attenuated vaccine is still not in widespread use. Here, by necessity, a comparatively rational approach to attenuation has been taken, which combines classical methods with contemporary genetics.

The second example, the polioviruses, represents one of the

major successes of live-attenuated vaccines. Since their introduction in the early 1960s, the Sabin oral polio vaccines have played a major role in reducing the incidence of paralytic poliomyelitis over much of the world. In spite of this, the molecular basis of attenuation of these strains is still not clear, but is a subject under intense investigation. This section reports on some of the latest findings in this area.

A. Influenza

1. Introduction and Pathogenicity Studies Influenza epidemics occur, as a result of antigenic changes in the virus surface glycoproteins, once every 2–3 years (for reviews, see Ward, 1981; Webster *et al.*, 1982). Over the past decade outbreaks have been relatively mild, causing only modest increases in morbidity and mortality. Occasionally however, as in 1957 (the H2N2 subtype) and 1968 (H3N2), there are major world-wide pandemics resulting from a major antigenic change of the haemagglutinin glycoprotein (anti-genic-shift). These have more serious consequences for public health. Indeed, workers in this area have drawn attention to the possibility of a pandemic similar in ferocity to that experienced in 1918–1919 in which an estimated 20 million people died (see Webster *et al.*, 1982).

Faced with the potential danger and the rapid global spread of new influenza epidemics, the classical approach to attenuation of the causative strain by protracted multiple passages in a foreign host seems extremely tenuous. Notwithstanding projected ideals of a universal influenza vaccine (Air *et al.*, 1980), antigenic variation means that a new vaccine needs to be developed against each new epidemic strain. Furthermore, the speed at which these epidemics spread through the community demands that a vaccine be available quickly if it is to be effective in preventing gross morbidity and mortality (Murphy *et al.*, 1976a). Therefore, efforts have been made to be prepared for any new epidemic. The aim is to have at our disposal the means to rapidly and confidently attenuate a wild disease-causing strain by a single-step method *in vitro*.

The influenza virus genome consists of eight distinct segments of single-stranded RNA ranging in size from 890 to 2400 nucleotides (for reviews see Palese, 1977; Scholtissek, 1978). Each RNA segment codes for at least one protein. Virus-coded proteins include three large polymerase (P) proteins, nucleocapsid protein (NP), at least three nonstructural proteins, a matrix protein, and two antigenically important surface glycoproteins against which virus neutralizing antibodies are directed—the haemagglutinin (HA) and neuraminidase (NA) (Palese, 1977; Almond and Barry, 1979; Scholtissek, 1978; Inglis and Almond, 1980; Lamb et al., 1981). The RNA segments possess a capacity to undergo genetic reassortment in a mixed infection so that progeny virions from a two-parent cross can theoretically form 256 (2^8) recombinant (reassortant) genetic types with equal frequency. Reassortment of RNA segments of human strains of virus with those of influenza A viruses from birds and mammals probably gives rise to antigenic shift (see Ward, 1981). Fortunately, reassortment also provides a potential means to rapidly attenuate any new strain (Kilbourne, 1969). The basic scheme is illustrated in Fig. 1. Essentially, it should be possible to diminish the disease-causing potential of any wild-type strain by reassortment of its genes with a well-characterized attenuated master strain. Thus, a candidate vaccine recombinant would derive its genes coding for the major antigenic determinants (HA and NA) from the wild strain and its remaining genes, including the ones carrying attenuating mutations, from the master strain.

It is self-evident that in this approach the pathogenicity of the wild-type virus should not be determined solely by the properties of its haemagglutinin and neuraminidase genes. Although in the case of avian influenza viruses the cleavability of the HA strongly influences pathogenicity (Bosch et al., 1979), this has not been observed in human strains. Indeed, a very early observation in influenza virus genetics made by Burnet and colleagues in the 1950s and later confirmed by others is that the haemagglutination characteristics of a strain can segregate independently in a mixed infection from its capacity to cause disease (Burnet and Lind, 1955; Rott et al., 1979). Thus the scheme outlined in Fig. 1 could in principle be used with any epidemic causing strain. The aim also is to be able to predict the level of attenuation of a given recombinant with confidence, based on an analysis of its genome composition by one of the established methods such as gel electrophoresis (Palese and

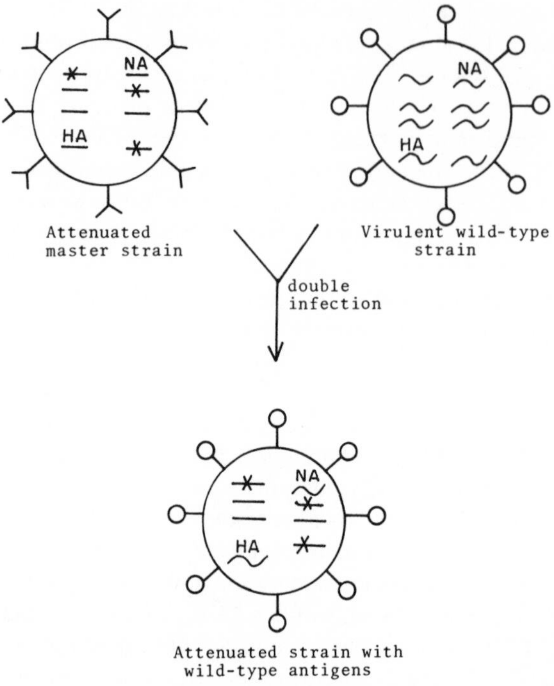

Fig. 1.　Use of gene reassortment to achieve attenuation of wild-type influenza virus. The eight individual genome segments can undergo reassortment in a mixed infection to give 256 (2^8) possible progeny types. The recombinant shown possesses the genome segments encoding the surface antigens (HA and NA) from the wild-type parent plus all six remaining segments from the attenuated master strain. X, hypothetical attenuating mutation.

Schulman, 1976; Almond *et al.*, 1977), hybridization (Scholtissek *et al.*, 1976), or by testing for the presence of identifiable genetic markers (Sugiura, 1975). Ideally the level of attenuation for humans should correlate well with results of simple laboratory tests, such as growth in tissue culture at different temperatures (Murphy *et al.*, 1976a), destruction of ciliated epithelia in tracheal organ cultures (Blaskovic *et al.*, 1972), or growth in small laboratory animals, such as hamsters (Friedewald and Hood, 1948) or ferrets (Basarab and Smith, 1969; Mills and Chanock, 1971). Suitable recombinants, following precedents derived from a variety of existing wild strains, would then ideally need only a limited trial in volunteers before being put into full scale production. It has been suggested that it may be possible under such circumstances, in the interests of speed, to license the attenuating process and the master strain, rather than the actual vaccine recombinant itself (Murphy *et al.,* 1976a; Schild *et al.,* 1976).

The major problem, therefore, becomes one of designing a master strain that will consistently donate the necessary qualities of attenuation to any recombinant. Unfortunately, so far, studies on pathogenicity have not provided a clear indication of precisely which genes determine or overwhelmingly influence pathogenicity and/or which genes must be modified to produce an acceptable level of attenuation. Results with the avian influenza, fowl plague virus (FPV), illustrate the problem. It was found that replacement of any of a number of single genes in a virulent strain (FPV-Rostock) with the corresponding gene from another strain of influenza virus could result in a complete loss of pathogenicity for chickens (Scholtissek *et al.,* 1977). However, loss of pathogenicity depends not only on the specific gene replaced but also on the strain from which the replacing gene is derived. Thus, if RNA segment 1 of FPV [coding for one of three polymerase proteins (P-tra) (Scholtissek, 1978)] is replaced by the corresponding gene from the laboratory adapted avirulent A/PR/8 strain, pathogenicity is completely lost. However, if the same RNA segment is derived from swine influenza virus, the recombinant is just as pathogenic as wild-type FPV/Rostock. Replacement of RNA segment 2 (coding for P1) with that from swine influenza on the other hand, results once again in complete loss of pathogenicity. Encouragingly, however, the general observation is that where more than one or two genes are derived from the apathogenic parent, a recombinant is likely to be less pathogenic than the wild-type. Nonetheless, exceptions are possible, for example: FPV recombinants possessing genes 1 and 2 from the human A/Hong Kong strain (apathogenic for chickens) had pathogenicity comparable to that of wild-type FPV. From these studies it was concluded that a specific gene or genes responsible for pathogenicity does not exist, but a certain gene constellation determines whether the recombinant virus is pathogenic or not (see Scholtissek, 1978; Rott, 1980).

Worrying observations that have a direct bearing on reassortment of genes as a means of attenuating influenza viruses have been made by Scholtissek and Vallbracht and colleagues. Recombinants neurovirulent for mice, which produce a generalized fatal infection involving the central nervous system, were obtained from genetic crosses in which neither of the parents possessed this property. In this case, the fowl influenza A/Avian/Rostock, mouse lung-adapted human strain A/England/1/61, and mouse pneumovirulent A/PR/8 were used (Vallbracht et al., 1979, 1980; Scholtissek et al., 1979). The properties of these recombinants were apparently the result of a gene constellation that neither parent possessed and could not have been predicted. Such results illustrate that caution is necessary when generating novel strains by gene reassortment, particularly when highly virulent avian strains are involved (see below).

Prior to and in spite of these findings, there have been a number of attempts to construct donor strains to provide a source of attenuating genes for genetic reassortment. Essentially, three different approaches have been used; the classical alternative host-adapted or host-range variant, temperature-sensitive mutants, and cold-adapted strains.

2. Host–Range Variants Passaging influenza virus many times in embryonated eggs has been used to produce host–range variants that grow poorly in man and do not cause symptoms of respiratory disease. This procedure however, is unpredictable and time-consuming. The number of passages required to sufficiently attenuate the virus may vary considerably from strain to strain and the time required can range from 3–9 months. Although this approach has been used by Russian workers for vaccine production more than thirty years ago (see Smorodincev, 1969), it was not until much later that attempts were made to use the attenuated strains in genetic reassortment (Beare and Hall, 1971; Beare et al., 1975). Recombinants between various epidemic strains and egg-adapted/attenuated A/Puerto Rico/8/34 or A/Okuda/57 have been produced and their level of attenuation assessed in human volunteers (McCahon et al., 1973, 1976). Recombinants of various degrees of virulence were obtained using either of these attenuated parents; some resembled the wild-type in the symptoms they caused, whereas others were considered safe enough to be tested as vaccines. Subsequently, many of the recombinants, especially of the A/PR/8 strain were analysed by gel electrophoresis to determine the parental origin of each of their genome segments in an attempt to show which genes from the avirulent or host-adapted parent correlated with an acceptable level of attenuation (Oxford *et al.,* 1978; Murphy *et al.,* 1980a). The results of this type of analysis led to the conclusion that it is not possible to predict the level of attenuation of a given recombinant solely by determining its genotype and that other factors, such as mutational events occurring during laboratory manipulations, probably play a role. Somewhat surprisingly, certain recombinants such as X-31 (derived from A/Aichi/68) (Beare *et al.,* 1975), which received all six of the transferable genes (i.e., those not coding for the surface antigens) from attenuated A/PR/8/34, retained a moderate virulence for man. Similar observations were obtained with an A/England/69 recombinant that received at least five of its genes from the A/PR/8 parent (Oxford *et al.,* 1978). The likely explanation of these observations is that, during the development of master strains by alternative host adaptation, mutations that contribute to the level of attenuation are acquired by the *HA* and *NA* genes. These genes are not inherited by the candidate vaccine recombinants. Indeed, one of the first changes occurring during passage in eggs which can be detected *in vitro,* the so-called O (original) to D (derived) change, involves alteration in haemagglutination characteristics (Burnet, 1955). This interpretation is also given credence by the finding that it is possible to further attenuate the recombinants themselves by selecting for a mutation in the haemagglutinin gene, manifested as resistance to serum inhibitors of haemagglutination (Lobmann *et al.,* 1976). However, mutations that demonstrably affect host–range, and probably thereby contribute to attenuation, certainly do occur in genes other than those encoding *HA* and *NA*. Thus the *P3* gene has been shown to be the site of mutation(s) involved in adaptation of an avian influenza strain A/FPV/Dobson to hamster kidney (BHK) and mouse L cells, although in this case capacity for replication in chick-embryo cells was undiminished (Almond, 1977; Almond and Barry, 1978). Mutations affecting host range have also been shown to occur elsewhere in the genome (Scholtissek and Murphy, 1978; Scholtissek *et al.,* 1978).

In summary, regular transfer of a predictable and satisfactory level of attenuation using the host-adapted master strains available to date has proved not to be straightforward. Recently, on the grounds that nature provides its own genetically stable alternative host-adapted strains that are avirulent for man (i.e., strains of influenza from other animals), it has been suggested that gene reassortment with avian influenza viruses could provide the basis for attenuation. Russian workers have produced recombinants using A/ FPV/Weybridge and suggested their use as candidate vaccines (Ghendon *et al.*, 1979). However, the results of Vallbracht *et al.* (1979) and Scholtissek *et al.* (1979) discussed in Section III,A,1 suggest that this could be positively dangerous.

   3. Temperature-Sensitive Mutants An initially promising approach to the attenuation of influenza viruses for vaccine purposes, making use of gene reassortment, has been pioneered by Chanock, Murphy, and colleagues at the National Institutes of Health, Bethesda, Maryland. The rationale involves the use of temperature-sensitive (*ts*) mutants attenuated for man (Mills and Chanock, 1971). In addition to being attenuated for reasons discussed in the previous section, mutants that are restricted in their replication *in vitro* at 37–38°C should be similarly limited in their capacity for growth in the human lower respiratory tract, the major site of significant pathology. Such mutants, however, should grow with reasonable efficiency in the cooler passages of the upper respiratory tract (32–34°C), giving rise to an infection that is mild or not apparent but is sufficient to stimulate local and systemic immunological defence mechanisms (Richman *et al.*, 1975; Murphy *et al.*, 1976a). The aim therefore is to develop master strains with well-characterized *ts* lesions and to be able to rapidly transfer the *ts* character to any new epidemic strain, thereby effecting a predictable degree of attenuation. In principle, *ts* mutations can affect any gene of the virus, and because any such mutation would limit virus growth in the warmer passages of the lower respiratory tract, and thereby inhibit pathological damage, its precise location within the genome may be unimportant. It is, of course, implicit that any *ts* master strain to be used in reassortment must not have its attenuating *ts* mutation(s) in the genes coding for the neuraminidase or haemagglutinin, because these would not be inherited by a candidate vaccine recombinant. An advantage of *ts* mutations is the ease with which their acquisition can be monitored *in vitro*. Plaque-formation or CPE assays at different temperatures are easy to perform and can readily be used for screening recombinants (Spring *et al.*, 1975a). Ideally, once the gene(s) carrying the *ts* lesion(s) have been transfered to a wild-type virus, any recombinant containing them should exhibit a predictable and consistent level of attenuation.

Murphy and colleagues have extensively evaluated two *ts* mutant master strains for their usefulness in facilitating attenuation of new antigenic variants. These are the A/Hong Kong/ts[1]E and A/Udorn/ts-1-A2.

In the case of ts[1]E, the genes carrying the *ts* mutations have been identified as RNA segment 1, encoding the polymerase protein P3, and RNA segment 5 encoding the nucleocapsid protein (NP) (Palese and Ritchey, 1977). Both of these proteins have a role in RNA synthesis in the infected cell (Palese, 1977; Scholtissek, 1978). ts[1]E, which has been investigated extensively by complementation analysis, was derived from a 5-flourouracil-induced mutant of A/Great Lakes/65 by recombination with A/Hong Kong/68 (Spring *et al.*, 1975b). Work has been aimed towards determining whether the level of attenuation provided by these *ts* mutations is acceptable and whether transfer to other subtypes is possible. This has been evaluated by testing A/Hong Kong/68-ts[1]E itself and ts[1]E recombinants possessing surface antigens of A/Udorn/72/ A/GA/74 and A/Victoria/75. Results in human volunteers suggested that, to be attenuated, a recombinant must possess both *ts* genes (*NP* and *P3*). The presence of only one *ts* gene in the recombinant was associated with an unacceptable level of illness. Evidence that it was the *ts* mutations *per se* that were responsible for attenuation was provided by the observation that substitution of wild-type genes for those of the ts[1]E attenuated donor parent at any locus other than those coding for *P3* and *NP* did not affect the level of attenuation of the resulting recombinant (Murphy *et al.*, 1980b; Markoff *et al.*, 1979). Challenge experiments using homologous wild-type virus revealed significant protection against disease (Murphy *et al.*, 1978a; Richman *et al.*, 1976). Furthermore, there was some epidemiological evidence (Wright *et al.*, 1977) that vaccination with A/Hong Kong/ts[1]E offered some protection against a related but heterologous natural infection with A/Port Chalmers/73. Such heterologous protection is not generally seen with inactivated vaccine.

Final analysis of results using ts[1]E-derived viruses, however, was disappointing. In volunteers lacking haemagglutination-inhibiting (HI) antibodies, but possessing antineuraminidase (NI) antibodies, the recombinants proved sufficiently attenuated. However, in doubly seronegative volunteers (i.e., HI and NI negative) the ts[1]E recombinants caused some febrile illness and were therefore not suitable as vaccines (Monto and Kendal, 1973; Murphy et al., 1980a). In addition, although earlier studies in adults had indicated the contrary (Murphy et al., 1976b), evidence of genetic instability after trials in children began to emerge. In some trials, virus that had lost the ts phenotype was recovered from 25% of the vaccinees (Wright et al., 1975; Kim et al., 1976). The final conclusion, therefore, was that ts[1]E genes were genetically insufficiently stable and too weakly attenuating for construction of recombinants to be used as vaccines in completely susceptible individuals (Murphy et al., 1980a). Murphy and colleagues therefore turned their attention to a second and more defective mutant ts-1-A2 (Murphy et al., 1978b).

ts-1-A2 was constructed from two ts mutants, both of which seemed to be genetically more stable and more defective than ts[1]E. These parent viruses were A/Udorn/72-ts-1A and A/Hong Kong/68-ts 314, both of which contained single ts lesions in the genes coding for polymerase proteins P1 and P3, respectively (Massicot et al., 1980a). These proteins are believed to play a role in early RNA synthesis in the infective cycle (Scholtissek, 1978). A recombinant derived from a genetic cross between these two mutants, designated A/Udorn/72 ts-1-A2 contained both the ts mutations (as determined by complementation tests), had a 37°C shut-off temperature (compared to 38°C for ts[1]E), and was more restricted for growth in both the upper and lower respiratory tract in experimental animals (Murphy et al., 1978a). Initial results with this mutant were encouraging. As with ts[1]E, the ts mutations could be transfered to wild-type viruses of alternative serotypes to bring about a consistent and predictable level of attenuation. ts-1-A2 derivatives of A/Victoria/3/75 (H3N2), A/Alaska/6/77 (H3N2), and A/Hong Kong/123/77 (H1N1) were prepared by gene reassortment (Murphy et al., 1978c,d, 1980a,b). All were significantly attenuated, illustrating once more that attenuation is effected by the presence of the ts mutations and hinting that the influence of other genes is minimal (Massicot et al., 1980b). Figure 2 shows results of virus replication in lungs and nasal turbinates of hamsters of ts-1-A2 recombinants. The virus essentially failed to grow in lungs

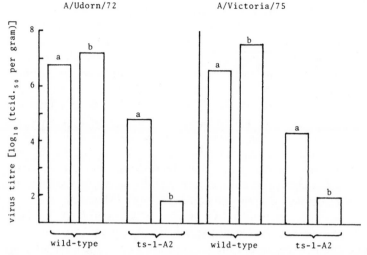

Fig. 2.   Viral replication in (a) the nasal turbinates and (b) the lungs of hamsters infected intranasally with 10 tcid$_{50}$ of Udorn/72 wild-type, Udorn/72-ts-1A2, Vic/75 wild-type, or Vic/75-ts-1A2 virus. Eight hamsters per virus were killed daily for 4 days, and the lungs and nasal turbinates were harvested. Each organ homogenate was titred individually, and the mean log$_{10}$ titres were determined for each day. The maximum level of replication achieved for each virus over the 4-day period is indicated. Redrawn from data provided by Murphy *et al.* (1978c).

and was restricted approximately 100-fold in its growth in nasal turbinates as compared to the wild-type. Initial observations on genetic stability in hamsters was similarly encouraging; no evidence of reversion to wild-type was observed (Murphy *et al.*, 1978c,d). In doubly seronegative human volunteers, a ts-1-A2 recombinant of A/Victoria/77 infected 90% of recipients causing only mild coryza or rhinitis in 5% of cases. Virus shedding was low, and the virus that was isolated seemed to have retained the ts phenotype. Challenge of vaccinees with wild-type virus revealed a significant level of protection (Murphy *et al.*, 1979a). However results with A/Hong Kong/77 recombinants sounded a note of caution. Although these viruses were significantly attenuated, there were one or two cases of febrile illness. More disturbingly genetic instability was observed with the A/Alaska/ts-1-A2 recombinants in some children with no previous experience of influenza. Furthermore, virus was shed for up to 10 days.

4. Cold Adaptation As discussed in the previous section, during the 1950s and early 1960s several researchers noticed an inverse relationship between the capacity of some viruses to cause disease and their ability to grow at low temperature. These observations, together with some early studies by Russian workers (Zdhanov, 1967), led Maassab to investigate cold adaptation as a method for attenuating influenza viruses. The approach was to combine the classical alternative host adaptation with growth at suboptimal temperature. Maassab worked initially with A/Ann Arbor/6/60 influenza virus and adapted this strain to growth at 25°C by gradually lowering the temperature of incubation over 20 passages in chicken kidney tissue culture followed by over 18 passages in the allantoic cavity of embryonated hens eggs (Maassab, 1967). The resulting cold-adapted (CA) strain (A/AA/6/60/CA), unlike its wild-type parent, replicated quite efficiently at 25°C in chicken kidney cells in tissue culture. A consequence of the cold-adaptation procedure is usually the development of a temperature-sensitive phenotype. A/AA/6/60/CA has a shut-off temperature for plaque formation of 37°C (Maassab *et al.*, 1969). This virus was initially tested in mice and ferrets and was found to be less pathogenic for these hosts than the wild-type non-CA parent (Maassab *et al.*, 1969). It became apparent also that, as with *ts* strains, not only was the A/AA/6/60/CA itself attenuated (Kitayama, 1973), but it also could be used as a donor of attenuating genes to epidemic influenza strains by gene reassortment (Maassab *et al.*, 1972). Thus cold-adapted versions of various subtypes, including A/Queensland/72, A/Dunnedin/73, A/Scotland/74, A/Victoria/75, A/Alaska/77, and A/Hong Kong/77, have been constructed, and some of these have been evaluated in human volunteers (Davenport *et al.*, 1977; Hrabar *et al.*, 1977; Reeve *et al.*, 1980; Murphy *et al.*, 1979b, 1980b;). Most cold recombinants were significantly attenuated although there were variations in reactogenicity between subtypes. If the CA phenotype was used as the sole genetic marker in the isolation of cold recombinants, variations in temperature sensitivity were observed (Spring *et al.*, 1978). However, these did not correlate directly with the level of attenuation (Murphy *et al.*, 1979b; 1980b; Maassab *et al.*, 1981). The results imply that mutations in genes other than those conferring the CA and *ts* phenotypes may contribute to the level of attenuation. Neither of these phenotypes can therefore be used as reliable indicators of attenuation *in vitro*. Previous genetic analyses on cold recombinants had suggested that the CA phenotype is a property conferred by at least three genes (Cox *et al.*, 1979). Recently, however, a careful analysis of cold recombinants prepared in MDCK cells at 33°C containing only single genes from the A/AA/6/60/CA parent have shown that the CA phenotype can be independently conferred by each of two genes, RNA segment 2 (encoding P1) and RNA segment 5 (encoding neuraminidase) (Odagiri *et al.*, 1982). In this study, the temperature-sensitive character was seen to be partially independent of the CA phenotype and was tentatively concluded to be a synergistic effect of mutations in genes 2 and 3. The finding that the *NA* gene can contribute to the CA phenotype is interesting but unfortunate, because this gene, by design, is not normally transferred to recombinants prepared for vaccine purposes.

General experiences with gene reassortment in relation to virus virulence (Oxford *et al.*, 1978) lends support to the view that mutations in other genes may contribute to the level of attenuation in cold-adapted strains. It is noteworthy that a non-*ts* non-CA attenuating mutation has been observed in a 5FU-induced *ts* mutant. This mutation segregated independently of the *ts* gene in a mixed infection (Richman *et al.*, 1977). The cold-adaptation regime involved multiple passages in chicken kidney cells, and it is likely that attenuating mutations of the host-adaptation type have occurred during this procedure. Further work is required to determine the individual and combined contributions of the *ts*, CA (and other mutations) of A/AA/6/60 CA to the level of attenuation of cold recombinants. Meanwhile cold recombinants, which derive all six of their transferable genes from the CA parent, can be considered good candidate vaccines (Maassab *et al.*, 1981). It is encouraging that under standard laboratory conditions for construction of cold recombinants (Cox *et al.*, 1979) more than 50% of isolates were of this type. Such recombinants can be constructed rapidly and are sufficiently attenuated even for use in young children (Wright *et al.*, 1982). Their genetic stability and low transmissibility render cold recombinants the most promising prospective live-attenuated influenza vaccines.

B. Poliomyelitis

1. Development of oral polio vaccines. Although introduced a few years later than inactivated polio vaccines (IPV), live-attenuated orally administered polio vaccines (OPV) have been adopted by many countries of the world and have played a significant role over the past two decades in causing a dramatic reduction in the incidence of paralytic poliomyelitis and in breaking the regular pattern of epidemics that had become familiar in the Western world during the first half of this century.

Polioviruses can be divided into three distinct serotypes, each of which is capable of causing paralytic disease in an estimated 1% of infected individuals. Because immunity to any one of these serotypes does not provide protection against the other two, vaccines must contain all three types. A major landmark heralding the possibility of developing live-attenuated vaccines against poliomyelitis was the propagation of the Lansing strain poliovirus in tissues of nonneural origin *in vitro* (Enders *et al.,* 1949). Encouraged by the results of Theiler with yellow fever and by the realization that a number of viruses affecting the nervous system may replicate in heterologous tissues *in vivo* (Evans and Chambers, 1948; Rustigian and Pappenheimer, 1949), several investigators attempted to develop, by various strategies, strains of poliovirus with reduced neurotropism. The race to production of an effective polio vaccine is an interesting tale but one that is well-recorded elsewhere (Sabin, 1965; Paul, 1971).

The attenuated polioviruses currently in use were developed by Sabin in the late 1950s. The precise details of the passage history *in vitro* and *in vivo,* leading to the attenuation of each of the three serotypes, is given in detail by Sabin and Boulger (1973) and, to clarify the discussion in the following section, is summarized in Fig. 3. The pattern was similar for serotypes 1 and 3, consisting of some 50 passages *in vitro* interspersed with about 20 passages *in vivo* in rhesus and cynomolgus monkeys. The most notable distinction between the three vaccines lies in the nature of the original isolates used. For serotypes 1 and 2, the original viruses (P1/Mahoney/41 and P2/P712/56) were isolated from the faeces of healthy children and thus were not directly associated with a case of human paralysis. In the case of serotype 2, the strain isolated was probably

Type 1
   P1/Mahoney/41   14 passages *in vivo* (monkeys)
     (Faecal isolate,   2 passages *in vitro* (monkey testicle)
     healthy children)

                         ↓

   P1/Mahoney/Monk14 T2   24 passages *in vitro* (monkey testicle)
                      18 passages *in vitro* (monkey kidney)
                      10 alternate passages:-
                       5 *in vivo* (intradermally in monkeys)
                       5 *in vitro* (monkey kidney)

                         ↓

   P1/Mahoney/Ls-c   5 passages *in vitro* (monkey kidney)
   Sabin (1956)   3 plaque purifications (monkey kidney)
                       2 passages *in vitro* (preparative) (monkey kidney)

   P1/Ls-c, 2ab/KP2/56
   Sabin vaccine strain.

Type 2
   P2/P712/56   4 passages *in vitro* (monkey kidney)
   Sabin (1956)   3 plaque purifications (monkey kidney)
     (Faecal isolate,   1 passage *in vivo* (orally in chimpanzees)
     healthy children)   3 plaque purifications (monkey kidney)

   P2/P712,Ch,2ab/KP2/56
   Sabin vaccine strain.

Type 3
   P3/Leon/37   21 passages *in vivo* (intracerebrally in monkeys)
     (Isolate from fatal   8 passages *in vitro* (monkey testicle)
     paralytic case)

                       ↓

   Sabin *et al.*   39 passages *in vitro* (monkey kidney)
   (1954)   3 plaque purifications (monkey kidney)
                       3 passages *in vitro* (preparative) (monkey kidney)
   P3/Leon 12a $_1$b KP3/56
   Sabin vaccine strain.

Fig. 3.   Derivation of the Sabin vaccine strains of poliovirus.

a naturally occurring variant of low neurovirulence for cynomolgus monkeys and was passaged fewer times than the type 1 or type 3 strains. In contrast, the original isolate of poliovirus type 3 (P3/ Leon/37) was isolated from the brain stem and spinal cord of a child that had suffered a fatal case of paralysis. These differences in the origin of the starting material may be significant in light of the figures now available on the incidence of vaccine associated disease (World Health Organization 1982). As mentioned earlier, strains isolated from cases of paralysis and designated "vaccine-like" are most commonly serotype 3 (World Health Organization 1982).

2. *The molecular basis of attenuation.* Parallel to the experiences gained with the use of oral polio virus, the past 20 years have also been a vast accumulation of knowledge on the molecular details of poliovirus structure and replication. Polioviruses are small icosahedral particles with a diameter of approximately 27 nm and are classified as members of the enterovirus genus of the family picornaviridae. They possess a single-stranded messenger-sense RNA genome of M_r 2.6×10^6 (approximately 7.5 kilobases), enclosed in a protein capsid composed of 60 copies of each of four virus coded polypeptides VP1, VP2, VP3, and VP4, ranging in M_r from 8 to 35 kilodaltons (Putnak and Philips, 1981). The replication of polioviruses, particularly the type 1 strain, P1/Mahoney, has received considerable attention mainly because it has been regarded as a prototype for viruses using this strategy of replication. Many details of the mechanisms of translation, processing, and RNA replication are now known (Rueckert, 1976; Perez-Bercoff, 1979; Kitamura *et al.*, 1981). In spite of this, however, the events responsible for the attenuation of Sabin's vaccine strains are still not precisely defined.

Early studies attempted to correlate physical properties of the virus particle with attenuation or virulence (Dubes and Wenner, 1957). For example, it was observed that the so-called *d* characteristic, which relates to efficiency of plating in cell culture under acid overlay medium, showed some correlation with the degree of neurovirulence (Vogt *et al.*, 1957). Other workers observed a differential affinity between attenuated and virulent strains for various compounds, such as calcium phosphate, cellulose resin, or aluminum hydroxide (Hodes *et al.*, 1960; Woods and Robbins, 1961; Wallis *et al.*, 1962; Koza, 1963). Differences have also been observed in the degree to which various strains aggregate in conditions of low ionic strength (Totsuka *et al.*, 1978). The P1/Sabin vaccine strain is more labile in the presence of SDS than the virulent P1/Mahoney strain from which it was derived (Young and Moon,

1975). These results suggest that attenuated strains have altered physical and particularly surface properties, a conclusion that is further strengthened by the finding that small antigenic differences exist between P1/Sabin and P1/Mahoney (Van Wezel and Hazendonk, 1979; Nakano *et al.*, 1978). This finding is concordant with the nucleotide sequence of the genomes of these two strains, as interpreted in the light of recent information on the location of a major antigenic site on the virus particle (Kitamura *et al.*, 1981; Racaniello and Baltimore, 1981a; Nomoto *et al.*, 1982; Minor *et al.*, 1983).

For none of the foregoing physical changes has it been possible to show a cause-and-effect relationship with attenuation. However, the possibility that attenuation involves physical changes to the surface of the virus particle has been an attractive model for some considerable time. Sabin suggested that the neurovirulence of a poliovirus may be determined by its specific interaction with neuronal target cells (Sabin, 1956). Mutations giving rise to a reduced affinity of the virus for nerve cells at the level of cell-receptor binding would thereby possess an attenuated phenotype. Such a model suggests that a difference may exist between virus recognition of cells of neural origin and of gut cells, because attenuated strains are perfectly capable of replication in the alimentary tract. At the present time, there is no evidence for such a difference.

The possibility that Sabin's vaccine strains are attenuated simply because they have acquired random *ts* mutations has been considered (Lwoff, 1959, 1969; Sabin, 1961). Certainly all the vaccine strains exhibit a reduced capacity for growth at 40°C. Such *ts* mutations could themselves affect the surface properties of the virus and thereby influence cell–virus interactions. However, it is interesting to note that there are reports of *ts* mutations in P1/Sabin, affecting later stages of the replication cycle, e.g., in translation of virus-specific RNA and in virus assembly (Denniston–Thompson and Tershak, 1976; Fiszman *et al.*, 1972).

In the last few years, it has become apparent that the approach most likely to discern meaningful differences between neurovirulent and attenuated strains is an analysis of virus nucleic acid. The technique of T1 oligonucleotide fingerprinting, having found wide application in strain differentiation and having provided strong evidence of vaccine-induced disease (Minor, 1980, 1982; Kew *et al.,* 1980), has been applied to a characterization of the genomes of the P1/Sabin vaccine strain and its neurovirulent progenitor, P1/ Mahoney (Nomoto *et al.,* 1981). This analysis revealed that no major changes in the genome, such as large insertions or deletions, had occurred. Only seven point mutations were detected, providing an estimate of 35 for the whole genome. In some cases, it was possible to define these mutations precisely by sequencing the altered oligonucleotides. However, as with the physical differences mentioned above, it has not been possible to correlate directly any of these with the attenuated phenotype. The results obtained have recently been verified but also superseded by a more detailed examination of virus genomes that offers to define precisely all differences that exist between neurovirulent and attenuated strains.

A major landmark in the study of the molecular biology of polioviruses was the publication by two laboratories almost simultaneously of the complete genome sequence of P1/Mahoney (Kitamura *et al.,* 1981; Racaniello and Baltimore, 1981a). As well as providing major new insights into the mechanisms of picornavirus replication, these studies have paved the way for exact comparisons of virulent and attenuated strains. Nomoto *et al.* (1982) have recently produced the total genome sequence of P1/Sabin and have thereby been able to catalogue all the mutations that occurred during its derivation from P1/Mahoney. Fifty-seven mutations, all single base substitutions, from a total of 7441 nucleotides, were observed. Twenty-one of these resulted in amino acid changes, which, although generally scattered throughout the genome, included 12 in the structural protein region. Five of these were clustered within 20 amino acids approximately in the middle of the virus protein VP1 (ringed in Fig. 4). This cluster appears a very likely candidate for the type of change that might support a model of attenuation based on the differential binding of virus to nerve and gut cells as discussed previously. Recent results from a collaborative study between our laboratory and NIBSC, London (Minor *et al.,* 1983), have a direct bearing on this interpretation. Making use of a panel of 16 different neutralizing monoclonal antibodies, it has been possible to isolate a large number of mutants of the P3/Leon strain possessing altered antigenicity. In an analysis similar to that used for influenza viruses (Yewdell and Gerhard, 1981), these mutants behave as 10 distinct but interdependent groups in their pattern of reaction with each of the monoclonal antibodies, favouring the conclusion that they possess alterations in different epitopes of a single major antigenic site. Nucleotide sequence analysis of representatives of 8 of the 10 groups of mutants suggests a location for this antigenic determinant at approximate amino acid positions 75 to 95 of virus protein VP1, (underlined in Fig. 4). Interestingly, this site is analogous to the location of the cluster of five amino-acid changes in VP1 of the P1/Sabin vaccine strain observed by Nomoto *et al.* (1982) mentioned above.

If one postulates that the basis of virus neutralization is inhibition, through antibody binding, of virus attachment to the host cell [indeed experimental evidence that this may be the case exists for at least some monoclonal antibodies (P.D. Minor, personal communication)], then it is reasonable to assume that the neutralizing-antibody binding site and the cell-receptor binding site may be spacially very close on the surface of the virus or may even be identical. The region defined by the monoclonal antibody study as the antigenic site may therefore be precisely the region of VP1 in which modifications having a differential effect on attachment to nerve and gut cells could be expected to be found. Thus the cluster of mutations observed in this region of VP1 could be those responsible for attenuation. However, there is an alternative explanation. Development of the P1/Sabin vaccine strain involved repeated passages by intradermal injection in rhesus or cynomolgus monkeys *in vivo* (see Fig. 3). During these passages, the virus would have encountered immune selection pressure, and, as a result, variants with altered antigenicity may have arisen. Such variants would of course be modified in the region of VP1 comprising the antigenic site. Thus the cluster of changes in VP1 of P1/Sabin could be due to antigenic changes that are totally independent of a mutation or mutations giving rise to attenuation. The results described below lend weight to this latter interpretation.

It may be significant that in contrast to the case of serotype 1, the 21 passages in monkeys during the attenuation of P3/Sabin were exclusively via the intracerebral route (see Fig. 3). At this location, the virus would not have encountered the same type and range of specific immune responses that the P1/Mahoney strain encountered during intradermal passage. We have therefore based our study of attenuation on serotype 3. Our results suggest that at least for this

POLIO TYPE 1 MAHONEY
POLIO TYPE 1 SABIN

POLIO TYPE 3 LEON
POLIO TYPE 3 LEON
POLIO TYPE 3 SABIN
POLIO TYPE 3 119

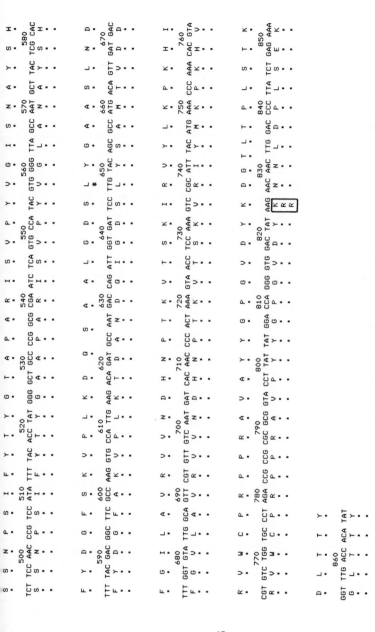

Fig. 4. Comparison of amino-acid sequence of the VP1 protein of virulent and attenuated strains of poliovirus. Data for P1/ Mahoney and P1/Sabin were taken from Racaniello and Baltimore (1981a) and Nomoto et al. (1982), respectively. Data for P3/Leon is from Minor et al. (1983). ○, amino acid sequence differences between virulent and attenuated type 1 strains. □, amino acid sequence differences between type 3 strains. The underlined region corresponds approximately to the antigenic site as defined by Minor et al. (1983).

45

serotype, the molecular basis of attenuation does not involve mutations in VP1. The three strains shown in Table I were chosen
because, in spite of possessing marked differences in neurovirulence in cynomolgus monkeys, they are identical serologically, they
induce infected-cell polypeptides indistinguishable from each other,
and their genomes produce identical T1 oligonucleotide finger-
prints. Therefore, there is a high probability that any observed
change in nucleotide sequence between these three strains might
relate directly to attenuation. P3/Leon/37 is the neurovirulent parent
of the P3/Sabin 12a₁b vaccine strain (see Fig. 3), and the strain
designated P3/119 is believed to be a neurovirulent revertant of the
vaccine strain, having been isolated from a fatal case of paralytic
poliomyelitis associated with vaccination (Minor, 1980). Any
mutations observed by comparing P3/Leon and P3/Sabin that relate
to attenuation are likely to have reverted to the parental form in the
genome of P3/119 (although suppressor mutations at distant sites
are also possible).

Molecular cloning of the genomes of plaque-purified isolates of
each of these three strains by an RNA·cDNA hybrid method (van
der Werf *et al.*, 1981; Cann *et al.*, 1983) has facilitated comparative
nucleotide sequencing studies. For reasons apparent from the previous discussion, initial effort has been directed towards the region
encoding VP1. These results are illustrated in Fig. 4. The similarity
in nucleotide sequence of the three type 3 strains was remarkably
high (the few changes are boxed in Fig. 4). Only a single base
difference between P3/Leon and P3/Sabin, out of the entire 867
nucleotides coding for VP1, was observed. This results in a chemically and structurally minor amino acid change of lysine to arginine
at amino acid position 274, well away from the cluster of mutations
observed in P1/Sabin and intuitively less of a change than that
which might be expected to account for attenuation. Furthermore,

TABLE I   Poliovirus Type-3 Strains

Strains	Process	Isolate number
P3/Leon/37	Virulent	970
P3/Sabin	Attenuated	411
P3/119	Virulent	643

this amino acid remains as arginine in the revertant P3/119, although one other change between this strain and P3/Sabin, towards the carboxy-terminus of the VP1 polypeptide (valine to alanine at position 43) has occurred. Although it is possible that these amino acid sequence changes could account for, or contribute to, attenuation and subsequent reversion to neurovirulence, their minor chemical nature and their disparate locations favours the conclusion that they do not. It appears, then, that the mutations responsible for attenuation in the P3/Sabin vaccine probably lie elsewhere in the genome. Further nucleotide sequencing is in progress, but whether this will provide a clear answer in the absence of a complementary genetic approach (Cooper, 1968; Racaniello and Baltimore, 1981b) remains to be seen.

These results do not rule out the possibility that changes in VP1 can result in attenuation and that this is the explanation in the case of the P1/Sabin vaccine. It is of course conceivable that the molecular basis of attenuation in each of the three Sabin vaccine strains may be completely different.

IV. CONCLUDING REMARKS

For most of the microorganisms for which live-attenuated vaccines have been developed to date, only a scant understanding exists of their mechanisms of pathogenesis. It has not usually been possible, therefore, to identify a particular pathogenicity factor as a target for modification or deletion. For attenuation through temperature-sensitive mutations this is perhaps unimportant, particularly since it seems that almost any *ts* lesion can cause a reduction in virulence irrespective of its location within the genome (see Richman *et al.*, 1975). However, a clear understanding of the molecular basis of attenuation of a microorganism by other means demands a parallel understanding of the molecular basis of its pathogenicity. It is axiomatic that research on attenuation will proceed hand in hand with research on microbial virulence mechanisms, and it is likely that, as our knowledge of these subjects increases, novel ways of attenuating microorganisms will become apparent. Blindly attenuated strains will continue to be useful in that they serve to illustrate those properties of a microorganism that are indispensible to its pathogenic character. However, in future, live-attenuated strains may be designed on more rational precepts.

An in-depth study of reoviruses by Fields and colleagues has recently provided an elegant illustration of the way in which research on the genetic and molecular mechanisms of pathogenesis, can contribute significantly to our understanding of attenuation (for a review see Fields and Green, 1982). Making use of the ability of reovirus to undergo genetic reassortment, it has been possible to decipher the individual contributions to pathogenicity in mice of several virus polypeptides. Modification of any one of these polypeptides can give rise to an attenuated virus. Thus, an alteration of the σ1 polypeptide, important in binding the virus to the host cell, can lead to reduced affinity for target cells and a modification of tissue tropism, thereby drastically affecting the course of disease (Spriggs and Fields, 1982; Fields and Green, 1982). Modification of the μ1c polypeptide may diminish the ability of the virus to establish infection via its natural oral route of entry to the body (Hrdy *et al.*, 1982). Finally, modification of the σ3 protein, believed to be involved in the inhibition of host RNA and protein synthesis, can lead to attenuation probably by affecting the ability of the virus to cause cell lysis (Fields and Green, 1982). Interestingly, strains continuously passaged in culture in a manner analogous to that used for vaccine development contained mutations in the gene encoding the σ3 protein (Mustoe *et al.*, 1978). Purposeful modification of the gene encoding this protein, for example, by the introduction of deletion mutations, may be a way in which this information could be used to produce very stable attenuated strains. It is important to note that the medically important rotaviruses fall within this family of viruses.

The induction of well-defined, stable mutations at predetermined sites within the genome may, therefore, be the way in which future live-attenuated vaccine strains are constructed. Already it has been proposed that a phosphonoacetic acid resistant, thymidine kinase negative mutant of herpes simplex virus be considered a candidate for vaccine use (Guari *et al.*, 1981). In this case, however, the proposal is probably premature, because much is yet to be learned about latency, neurotropism, and oncogenicity in these viruses. The recent results of Field and colleagues suggest that such mutants could possess sinister modifications of wild-type pathogenicity (Field *et al.*, 1982).

At first glance, it may seem that some of the newer technologies in biomedical sciences (see Chapters 3 and 4) could influence a movement away from attenuated strains towards a greater use of synthetic antigens. However, quite apart from concerns that first generation products of these methods may be inadequate immunogens (Kleid *et al.*, 1981), it is important to note that the new technologies may also provide a stimulus to the development of new methods of attenuation. There are now a number of examples where live animal viruses, even those containing RNA genomes, have been recovered from plasmid DNA vectors after cloning in *E. coli* (Peden *et al.*, 1980; Racaniello and Baltimore, 1981b). Similarly, particular regions of the genome of some pathogens have been cloned in *E. coli,* manipulated *in vitro,* and replaced into the parent organism (e.g., Post and Roizman, 1981; Shimotohno and Temin, 1981). Such studies offer exciting prospects for the study of microbial pathogenesis. They may also provide new ways of introducing stable attenuating mutations.

It is still the case that in all parts of the world infectious diseases pose major problems to human health. Drug therapy offers an inadequate long-term solution, and problems of resistance continue to increase. Vaccination is without doubt the best way to control these diseases. Attenuation is, and will continue to be, an important option in vaccine development.

REFERENCES

Air, G. M., Laver, W. G. and Webster, R. G. (1980). *In* "New Developments with Human and Veterinary Vaccines" (A. Mizrahi, I. Hertman, M. A. Klingberg and A. Kohn, eds.), pp. 193–215. Alan R. Liss, New York.

Almond, J. W. (1977). Nature *(London)* **270**, 617–618.

Almond, J. W. and Barry, R. D. (1978). *In* "Negative Strand Viruses and the Host Cell" (B. W. J. Mahy and R. D. Barry, eds.), pp. 675–684. Academic Press, New York.

Almond, J. W. and Barry, R. D. (1979). *Virology* **92**, 407–415.

Almond, J. W., McGeoch, D. and Barry, R. D. (1977). *Virology* **81**, 62–73.

Armstrong, C. (1929). *Pub. Health Rep. (USA)* **44**, 1183–1191.

Armstrong, C. and Lillie, R. D. (1929). *Pub. Health Rep. (USA),* 2635–2647.

Basarab, O. and Smith, H. (1969). *Br. J. Exp. Pathol.* **50**, 612–618.

Bazin, M. (1980). *Nature* (London) **285**, 7–8.

Baxby, D. (1981). "Jenner's Smallpox Vaccine." Heinemann, London.

Beare, A. S. and Hall, T. S. (1971). *Lancet* **ii**, 1271–1273.

Beare, A. S., Schild, G. C. and Craig, J. W. (1975). *Lancet* **ii**, 729–732.

Blaskovic, P., Rhodes, A. J. and Labzoffsky, N. A. (1972). *Arch. Gesamte Virus-forsch.* **37**, 104–113.

Bosch, F. X., Orlich, M., Klenk, H. D. and Rott, R. (1979). *Virology* **95**, 197–207.

Bunyak, E. B. and Hilleman, M. R. (1966). *Proc. Soc. Exp. Biol. Med.* **123**, 768–775.

Bunyak, E. B. Hilleman, M. R., Weibel, R. E. and Stokes, J. Jr. (1968). *J. Am. Med. Assoc.* **204**, 195–200.

Burgastow, P. N., Andzaparidze, O. G. and Popov, V. (1973). *Bull. W. H. O.* **49**, 571.

Burge, B. W. and Pfefferkorn, E. R. (1966). *Virology* **30**, 214–223.

Burnet, F. M. (1955). *In* "Principles of Animal Virology." Academic Press, New York.

Burnet, F. M. and Lind, P. E. (1955). *Aust. J. Exp. Biol. Med. Sci.* **33**, 281–295.

Buxton, A. and Fraser, G. (1978). "Animal Microbiology." Blackwell, Oxford.

Cann, A. J., Stanway, G., Hauptmann, R., Minor, P. D., Schild, G. C., Clarke, L. D., Mountford, R. C. and Almond, J. W. (1983). *Nucl. Acids Res.* **11**, 1267–1281.

Chanock, R. M. and Richman, D. D. (1975). *In* "Viral Immunology & Immunopath-ology," pp. 291–316. Academic Press, New York.

Cherry, J. D., Feigen, R. D., Lober, L. A. Jr. and Shackelford, P. G. (1972). *J. Pediat.* **50**, 712–717.

Churchill, A. E., Chubb, R. C. and Baxendale, W. (1969a). *J. Gen. Virol.* **4**, 557–564.

Churchill, A. E., Payne, L. N. and Chubb, R. C. (1969b). *Nature (London)* **221**, 744.

Cooper, P. D. (1964). *Virology* **22**, 186–192.

Cooper, P. D. (1968). *Virology* **35**, 584–596.

Cossart, Y. (1977), *Br. Med. J.* **1**, 1621–1623.

Cox, N. J., Maassab, A. J. and Kendal, A. P. (1979). *Virology* **97**, 190–194.

Davenport, F. M., Hennessy, A. V., Maassab, H. F., Minuse, E., Clark, L. C., Abrams, G. D. and Mitchell, J. R. (1977). *J. Infect. Dis.* **136**, 17–25.

Denniston-Thompson, K. and Tershak, D. R. (1976). *J. Mol. Biol.* **106**, 55–74.

Dubes, G. R. and Chapin, M. (1956). *Science* **124**, 586–588.

Dubes, G. R. and Wenner, H. A. (1957). *Virology* **4**, 275–296.

Elek, S. D. and Stern, H. (1974). *Lancet* **i**, 1–5.

Enders, J. F., Weller, T. H. and Robbins, F. C. (1949). *Science* **109**, 85–87.

Enders, J. F., Katz, S. L., Milovanovic, M. V. and Holloway, A. (1960). *N. Engl. J. Med.* **263**, 153–159.

Evans, C. A. and Chambers, V. C. (1948). *Proc. Soc. Exp. Biol. Med.* **68**, 436–442.

Fenner, F. and Cairns, J. (1959). *In* "The Viruses" (F. M. Burnet and W. N. Stanley, eds.), pp. 225–250. Academic Press, New York.

Field, H. J., Anderson, J. R. and Wildy, P. (1982). *J. Gen. Virol.* **59**, 91–99.

Fields, B. N. (1972). *New Engl. J. Med.* **287**, 1026–1033.

Fields, B. N. and Greene, M. I. (1982). *Nature (London)* **300**, 19–23.

Fiszman, M., Reynier, M., Bucchini, D. and Girrard, M. (1972). *J. Virol.* **10**, 1143–1151.

Fried, M. (1965). *Virology* **25**, 669–671.

Friedewald, W. F. and Hook, E. W. (1948). *J. Exp. Med.* **88**, 343.

Fulginiti, V. A. and Arthur, J. H. (1969). *J. Pediat.* **75**, 609–616.

Gauri, K. K., Schenk, K. D. and Pressler, K. (1981). *In* "Antiviral Chemotherapy Design of Inhibitors of Viral Functions" (K. R. Gauri, ed.), pp. 321–326. Academic Press, New York.

Ghendon, Y. Z., Marchenko, A. T., Markushin, S. G., Ghenkina, D. B. and Mikhejeva, A. V. (1973). *Arch. Ges. Virusforsch.* **42**, 154–159.

Ghendon, Y., Kilmov, A., Blagoveshenskaya, O. and Ghenkina, D. (1979). *J. Gen. Virol.* **43**, 183–191.

Harris, R. W., Isacson, P. and Karzon, D. T. (1969). *J. Pediat.* **74**, 552–563.

Hodes, A. L., Zepp, H. D. and Ainbender, E. (1960). *Virology* **11**, 306–308.

Hozinski, V. I., Seibel, V. B., Pantelyeva, N. S., Mazurova, S. M. and Novikova, E. A. (1966). *Acta Virol.* **10**, 20.

Hrabar, A., Vodopija, I., Andres, F. E., Mitchell, J. R., Maassab, H. F., Hennessy, A. V. and Davenport, F. M. (1977). *Dev. Biol. Stand.* **39**, 53–60.

Hrdy, D. B., Rubin, D. H. and Fields, B. N. (1982). *Proc. Natl. Acad. Sci. U.S.A.* **79**, 1298–1302.

Huygelen, C. (1978). *In* "New Trends and Developments in Vaccines" (A. Voller and H. Friedman, eds.), pp. 103–115. Academic Press, New York.

Huygelen, C. and Peetermans, J. (1967). *Arch. Ges. Virusforsch.* **21**, 357.

Inglis, S. C. and Almond, J. W. (1980). *Phil. Trans. R. Soc. London* **B288**, 375–381.

Isacson, P. and Stone, A. (1971). *Prog. Med. Virol.* **13**, 239.

Kapikian, A. Z., Mitchell, R. H. and Chanock, R. M. (1969). *Am. J. Epidemiol.* **89**, 405–421.

Kew, O. M., Pallansch, M. A., Omilianovoski, D. R. and Rueckert, R. R. (1980). *J. Virol.* **33**, 256–263.

Kilbourne, E. D. (1969). *Bull. W. H. O.* **41**, 643–651.

Kilham, L. (1959). *In* "Perspectives in Virology" (M. Pollard, ed.), pp. 54–62. Wiley, New York.

Kim, H. W., Canchola, J. G., Brandt, C. D., Pyles, G., Chanock, R. M., Jelson, K. E. and Parrott, R. H. (1969). *Am. J. Epidemiol.* **80**, 422–434.

Kim, H. W., Arrobio, J. O., Brandt, C. D., Parrott, R. H., Murphy, B. R., Richman, D. D. and Chanock, R. M. (1976). *Pediat. Res.* **10**, 238–242.

Kitamura, N., Semler, B. L., Rothberg, P. G., Larsen, G. R., Adler, C. J., Dorner, A. J., Emini, E. A., Hanecak, R., Lee, J. J., van der Werf, S., Anderson, C. W. and Wimmer, E. (1981). **291**, 547–553.

Kitayama, T., Yogo, Y., Hornick, R. B. and Friedwald, W. I. (1973). *Infect. Immunol.* **7**, 119–122.

Kleid, D. G., Yansura, D., Small, B., Dowbenko, D., Moore, D. M., Grubman, M. J., McKercher, P., Morgan, D. O., Robertson, B. H. and Bachrach, H. L. (1981). *Science* **214**, 1125–1129.

Koprowski, H. and Lennette, E. H. (1946). *J. Exp. Med.* **84**, 205–210.

Koza, J. (1963). *Virology* **21**, 477–481.

Lamb, R. A., Lai, C.-J. and Choppin, P. W. (1981). *Proc. Natl. Acad. Sci. U.S.A.* **78**, 4170–4174.

Langer, W. L. (1976). *Sci. Am.* **234**, 112–117.

Lobmann, M., Delen, A., Peetermans, J. and Huygelen, C. (1976). *J. Hyg. Camb.* **77**, 181–188.

Lwoff, A. (1959). *Bacteriol. Rev.* **23**, 109–124.

Lwoff, A. (1969). *Bacteriol. Rev.* **33**, 390–403.

Maassab, H. F. (1967). *Nature (London)* **213**, 612–614.

Maassab, H. F., Francis, T. Jr., Davenport, F. M., Hennessy, A. V., Minuse, E. and Anderson, G. (1969). *Bull. W. H. O.* **41**, 589–594.

Maassab, H. F., Kendall, A. P. and Davenport, F. M. (1972). *Proc. Soc. Exp. Biol. Med.* **139**, 768–773.

Maassab, H. F., DeBorde, D. C., Cox, N. J. and Kendal, A. P. (1981). *In* "Genetic Variation among Influenza Viruses" (D. Nayak, ed.), pp. 617–638. Academic Press, New York.

McCahon, D., Schild, G. C., Beare, A. S. and Hall, T. S. (1973). *Postgrad. Med. J.* **49**, 195–199.

McCahon, D., Beare, A. S. and Stealey, V. (1976). *Postgrad. Med. J.* **52**, 389–394.

Mackenzie, J. S. (1970). *J. Gen. Virol.* **6**, 63–75.

Markoff, L. J., Thierry, F., Murphy, B. R. and Chanock, R. M. (1979). *Infect. Immunol.* **26**, 280–286.

Markushin, S. G. and Ghendon, Y. Z. (1973). *Acta Virol.* **17**, 369–376.

Massicot, J. G., Murphy, B. R., Thierry, F., Markoff, L., Huang, K.-Y. and Chanock, R. M. (1980a). *Virology* **101**, 242–249.

Massicot, J. G., Murphy, B. R., Van Wyke, K., Huang, K.-Y. and Chanock, R. M. (1980b). *Virology* **106**, 187–190.

Melnick, J. L., Hsiung, G. D., Rappaport, C., Howes, D. and Reissing, M. *Tex. Rep. Biol. Med.* **15**, 532–533.

Mills, J. V. and Chanock, R. M. (1971). *J. Infect. Dis.* **123**, 145–157.

Mills, J., Chanock, R. M. and Alling, D. W. (1969). *Br. Med. J.* **4**, 690.

Minor, P. D. (1980). *J. Virol.* **34**, 73–84.

Minor, P. D. (1982). *J. Gen. Virol.* **59**, 307–317.

Minor, P. D., Schild, G. C., Bootman, J., Evans, D. M. A., Ferguson, M., Reeve, P., Spitz, M., Stanway, G., Cann, A. J., Hauptmann, R., Clarke, L. D., Mountford, R. C. and Almond, J. W. (1983). *Nature (London)* **301**, 674–679.

Monto, A. S. and Kendall, A. P. (1973). *Lancet* **i**, 623–625.

Moritz, A. J., Kunz, C., Hofman, H., Liehl, E., Reeve, P. and Maassab, H. F. (1980). *J. Infect. Dis.* **142**, 857–860.

Murphy, B. R., Spring, S. G. and Chanock, R. M. (1976a). *In* "Influenza Viruses, Vaccines and Strategy" (P. Selby, ed.), pp. 179–197. Academic Press, New York.

Murphy, B. R., Richman, D. D., Spring, S. B. and Chanock, R. M. (1976b). *Postgrad. Med. J.* **52**, 381–388.

Murphy, B. R., Markoff, L. J., Hosier, N. T., Rutsen, H. J., Chanock, R. M., Kendal, A. P., Douglas, R. G., Betts, R. F., Cate, Jr., T. R., Couch, R. B., Levine, M. M., Waterman, D. H. and Holley, Jr., H. P. (1978a). *Infect. Immunol.* **20**, 671–677.

Murphy, B. R., Wood, F. T., Massicot, J. G. and Chanock, R. M. (1978b). *Virology* **88**, 231–243.

Murphy, B. R., Wood, F. T., Massicot, J. G. and Chanock, R. M. (1978c). *Virology* **88**, 244–251.

Murphy, B. R., Hosier, N. T., Spring, S. B., Mostow, S. R. and Chanock, R. M. (1978d). *Infect. Immunol.* **20**, 665–670.

Murphy, B. R., Chanock, R. M., Levine, M. M., Van-Blerk, G. A., Berquist, E. J.,

Douglas, R. G., Betts, R. F., Couch, R. B. and Cate, Jr., T. R. (1979a). *Infect. Immunol.* **23**, 249–252.

Murphy, B. R., Holly, H. P., Berquist, E. J., Levine, M. M., Spring, S. B., Maassab, H. F., Kendal, A. P. and Chanock, R. M. (1979b). *Infect. Immunol.* **23**, 253–259.

Murphy, B. R., Markoff, L. J., Chanock, R. M., Spring, S. B., Maassab, H. F., Kendal, A. P., Cox, N. J., Levine, M. M., Douglas, Jr., R. G., Betts, R. F., Couch, R. B. and Cate, T. R., Jr. (1980a). *Phil. Trans. R. Soc. London* **B288**, 401–415.

Murphy, B. R., Margret, B. R., Gordon, Jr., R. D., Betts, R. F., Couch, R. B., Cate, Jr., T. R., Chanock, R. M., Kendal, A. P., Maassab, H. F., Suwanagool, S., Sotman, S. B., Cisneros, L. A., Anthony, W. C., Nalin, D. R. and Levine, M. M. (1980b). *Infect. Immunol.* **29**, 348–355.

Mustoe, T. A., Ramig, R. F., Sharpe, A. H. and Fields, B. N. (1978). *Virology* **85**, 545–556.

Nakano, J. H., Hatch, M. H., Thieme, M. L., and Nottay, B. (1978). *Prog. Med. Virol.* **24**, 178–206.

Nomoto, A., Kitamura, N., Lee, J. J., Rothberg, P. H., Imura, N. and Wimmer, E. (1981). *Virology* **112**, 217–227.

Nomoto, A., Omata, T., Toyoda, H., Kuge, S., Horie, H., Kataoda, Y., Genba, Y., Nakano, Y. and Imura, N. (1982). *Proc. Natl. Acad. Sci. U.S.A.* **79**, 5793–5797.

Norrby, E. (1975). *J. Biol. Stand.* **3**, 375.

Norrby, E. and Lagercrantz, R. (1976). *Acta Paed. Scand.* **54**, 171.

Norrby, E., Enders-Ruckle, G. and terMeulen, V. (1975). *J. Infect. Dis.* **132**, 262.

Odagiri, T., DeBorde, D. C. and Maassab, H. F. (1982). *Virology* **119**, 82–95.

Oduntan, S., Olu, S., Lucas, A. O. and Wennen, E. M. (1978). *Ann. Trop. Med. Parisitol.* **72**(2), 116.

Oxford, J. S., McGeoch, D. J., Schild, G. C. and Beare, A. S. (1978). *Nature (London)* **273**, 778–779.

Palese, P. (1977). *Cell* **10**, 1–10.

Palese, P. and Ritchey, M. (1977). *Virology* **78**, 183–191.

Palese, P. and Schulman, J. L. (1976). *J. Virol.* **17**, 876–884.

Parkman, P. D., Meyer, Jr., H. M., Kirschstein, R. L. and Hopps, H. E. (1966). *New Engl. J. Med.* **275**, 569–574.

Paul, J. R. (1971). "A History of Poliomyelitis." Yale Univ. Press, New Haven and London.

Peden, K. W. C., Pipas, J. M., Pearson-White, S. and Nathans, D. (1980). *Science* **209**, 1392–1396.

Perez-Bercoff (ed.) (1979). "The Molecular Biology of Picornaviruses." NATO Advanced Study Institutes Series A. Life Sciences, No. 23. Plenum, New York and London.

Plotkin, S. A., Farquhar, J., Katz, M. and Ingalls, T. H. (1967). *Am. J. Epidemiol.* **86**, 468–477.

Post, L. E. and Roizman, B. (1981). *Cell* **25**, 227–232.

Potash, L., Lees, R. S., Greenberger, J. L., Hoyrup, A., Denney, L. D. and Chanock, R. M. (1970). *J. Infect. Dis.* **121**, 640–647.

Provost, P. J., Franklyn, S. B., Giesa, P. A., McAleer, W. J., Bunyak, E. B. and Hilleman, M. R. (1982). *Proc. Soc. Exp. Biol. Med.* **170**, 8–14.

Purchase, H. G. (1976). *Cancer Res.* **36**, 696.

Putnak, J. R. and Philips, B. A. (1981). *Microbiol. Rev.* **45**, 287–315.

Rancaniello, V. R. and Baltimore, D. (1981a). *Proc. Nat. Acad. Sci. U.S.A.* **78**, 4887–4891.

Racaniello, V. R. and Baltimore, D. (1981b). *Science* **214**, 916–919.

Reeve, P., Almond, J. W., Felsenreich, V., Pibermann, M. and Maassab, H. F. (1980). *J. Infect. Disease* **142**, 850–856.

Richman, D. D., Murphy, B. R., Spring, S. B., Coleman, M. T. and Chanock, R. M. (1975). *Virology* **66**, 551–561.

Richman, D. D., Murphy, B. R., Chanock, R. M., Gwalthey, J. M., Douglas, R. G., Betts, R. F., Blacklow, N. R., Rose, F. B., Parrino, T. A., Levine, M. M. and Caplan, E. S. (1976). *J. Infect. Dis.* **134**, 585–594.

Richman, D. D., Murphy, B. R. and Chanock, R. M. (1977). *Virology* **83**, 356–364.

Rohitayodhin, S. and Hammon, W. (1962). *J. Immunol.* **89**, 589–597.

Rott, R. (1979). *Arch. Virol.* **59**, 285–298.

Rott, R. (1980). *Phil. Trans. R. Soc. London* **B288**, 393–399.

Rueckert, R. R. (1976). *In* "Comprehensive Virology" H. Fraenkel-Conrat and R. R. Wagner, eds.), pp. 131–213. Plenum, New York.

Rustigian, R. and Pappenheimer, A. M. (1949). *J. Exp. Med.* **89**, 69–92.

Sabin, A. B. (1956). *Science* **123**, 1151–1157.

Sabin, A. B. (1961). *In* "Perspectives in Virology" (M. Pollard, ed.), pp. 90–110. Raven, New York.

Sabin, A. B. (1965). *J. Am. Med. Assoc.* **194**, 872–876.

Sabin, A. B. and Boulger, L. (1973). *J. Biol. Stand.* **1**, 115–118.

Salk, J. and Salk, D. (1978). *In* "New Trends and Developments in Vaccines" (A. Voller and H. Friedman, eds.). MTP Press, England.

Schild, G. C., Oxford, J. S. and Wood, J. M. (1976). *In* "Influenza: Virus, Vaccines and Strategy" (P. Selby, ed.), pp. 227–243. Academic Press, New York.

Scholtissek, C. (1978). *Curr. Top. Microbiol. Immunol.* **80**, 139–169.

Scholtissek, C. and Murphy, B. R. (1978). *Arch. Virol.* **58**, 323–333.

Scholtissek, C., Harms, E., Rohde, W., Orlich, M. and Rott, R. (1976). *Virology* **74**, 332–344.

Scholtissek, C., Rott, R., Orlich, M., Harms, E. and Rhode, W. (1977). *Virology* **81**, 74–80.

Scholtissek, C., Koennecke, I. and Rott, R. (1978). *Virology* **91**, 79–85.

Scholtissek, C., Vallbracht, A., Flehmig, B. and Rott, R. (1979). *Virology* **95**, 492–500.

Selimov, M. A. and Nikitina, L. F. (1970). *Vop. Virusol.* **15**, 161–165.

Shimotohno, K. and Temin, H. M. (1981). *Cell* **26**, 67–77.

Smith, H., Skehel, J. J. and Turner, M. J. (eds.). (1980). "The Molecular Basis of Microbial Pathogenicity," pp. 1–355. Verlag Chemie, Basel.

Smorodincev, A. A. (1969). *Bull. W. H. O.* **41**, 585–588.

Spriggs, D. and Fields, B. N. (1982). *Nature (London)* **297**, 68–70.

Spring, S. B., Nusinoff, S. B., Tierney, E. L., Richman, D. D., Murphy, B. R. and Chanock, R. M. (1975a). *Virology* **66**, 542–550.

Spring, S. B., Nusinoff, S. R., Mills, J., Douglas, V., Richman, D., Tierney, E. L., Murphy, B. R. and Chanock, R. M. (1975b). *Virology* **66**, 522–532.

Spring, S. B., Maassab, H. F., Kendal, A. P., Murphy, B. R. and Chanock, R. M. (1978). *Arch. Virol.* **55**, 233–246.

Steele, J. H. (1975). *In* "The Natural History of Rabies" (G. M. Baer, ed.), pp. 1–29. Academic Press, New York.

Sugiura, A. (1975). *In* "The Influenza Viruses and Influenza" (E. D. Kilbourne, ed.). Academic Press, New York.

Sweet, B. H. and Hilleman, M. R. (1960). *Proc. Soc. Exp. Biol. Med.* **105**, 420–427.

Takahashi, M., Otsuka, T., Okuno, Y., Asano, Y., Yazaki, T. and Isomura, S. (1974). *Lancet* **ii**, 1288–1290.

Theiler, M. and Smith, H. H. (1937). *J. Exp. Med.* **65**, 767–787.

Totsuka, A., Ohtaki, K., and Tagaya, I. (1978). *J. Gen. Virol.* **38**, 519–533.

Vallbracht, A., Flehmig, B. and Gerth, H. J. (1979). *Intervirology* **11**, 16–22.

Vallbracht, A., Scholtissek, C. Flehmig, B. and Gerth, H. J. (1980). *Virology* **107**, 452–460.

Van der Werf., S., Bregegere, F., Kopecka, H., Kitamura, N., Rothberg, P. G., Kourilsky, P., Wimmer, E. and Girard, M. (1981). *Proc. Natl. Acad. Sci. U.S.A.* **78**, 5983–5987.

Van Wezel, A. L. and Hazendonk, A. G. (1979). *Intervirology* **11**, 2–8.

Vogt, M., Dulbecco, R. and Wenner, H. A. (1957). *Virology* **4**, 141–155.

Wagner, R. R. (1974). *Infect. Immunol.* **10**, 309–315.

Wallis, C., Melnick, J. L., Ferry, G. D. and Wimberly, I. L. (1962). *J. Exp. Med.* **115**, 763–775.

Ward, C. W. (1981). *Curr. Top. Microbiol. Immunol.* **94**, 1–74.

Webster, R. G., Laver, W. G., Air, G. M. and Schild, G. C. (1982). *Nature (London)* **296**, 115–121.

Weller, T. H. and Neva, F. A. (1962). *Proc. Soc. Exp. Biol. Med.* **11**, 215–224.

World Health Organization (1969). *Bull. W. H. O.* **40**, 925–945.

World Health Organization (1981). *Tech. Rep. Ser.* No. 658, 65.

World Health Organization (1982). *Bull. W. H. O.* **60**, 231–2242.

Witte, J. J. and Axnick, N. W. (1975). *Pub. Health Rep.* **90**, 205.

Woods, W. A. and Robbins, F. C. (1961). *Proc. Natl. Acad. Sci. U.S.A.* **47**, 1501–1507.

Wright, P. F., Woodend, W. G. and Chanock, R. M. (1970). *J. Infect. Dis.* **122**, 501–512.

Wright, P. F., Sell, S. H., Shinozaki, T., Thompson, J. and Karzon, D. T. (1975). *J. Pediat.* **87**, 1109–1116.

Wright, P. F., Shinovaki, T., Fleet, W., Sell, S. H., Thompson, J. and Karzon, D. T. (1976). *J. Pediat.* **88**, 931–936.

Wright, P. F., Ross, K. B., Thompson, J. and Karzon, D. T. (1977). *N. Engl. J. Med.* **296**, 829–834.

Wright, P. F., Okabe, N., McKee, K. T., Maassab, H. F. and Karzon, D. T. (1982). *J. Infect. Dis.* **146**, 71–79.

Yewdell, J. W. and Gerhard, W. (1981). *Annu. Rev. Microbiol.* **35**, 185–206.

Young, N.A. and Moon, R. J. (1975). *In Proc. 3rd Int. Congr. Virol.* (H. S. Bedson, R. Najerá, L. Valenciano, and P. Wildy, eds.), *International Association of Microbiological Societies*.

Zhdanov, V. M. (1967). *Proc. 1st Int. Conf. Vaccines against Viral and Rickettsial Diseases of Man Washington D.C. Pan American Health Organization Scientific Publication* No. 147, pp. 9–15.

Zygraich, N. and Huygelen, C. (1973). *Arch. Virusforsch* **43,** 103–111.

Zygraich, N., Lobmann, M. and Huygelen, C. (1972). *J. Hygiene* **70,** 229–234.

3

Gene Cloning in Vaccine Research

T. J. R. HARRIS

Celltech Ltd.
Slough, England

I. INTRODUCTION

There are several reasons why recombinant DNA techniques have been applied to vaccine research. Despite the successes of the smallpox and poliovirus vaccination programmes and the efficacy

IMMUNE INTERVENTION

of various bacterial vaccines (e.g., diphtheria), there are still several diseases of virus, bacterial, or parasite origin for which no satisfactory vaccine is available. Gene cloning not only provides the means for obtaining a greater understanding of the structure and replication of microorganisms, but it also offers novel ways of synthesising protein antigens. Although the recent commercial trends have been away from vaccines, the level of academic interest in novel approaches to vaccines has never been higher. This is not only because of the inherent interest and social importance of vaccines but also because recombinant DNA techniques developed from a combination of bacterial genetics and molecular virology. One of the reasons that the molecular biology of viruses was investigated was because it provided one of the best ways of probing the complex mechanisms of eukaryotic gene expression. With the availability of cloning methods for doing this, the emphasis has shifted back to the viruses themselves and to the vaccines against them.

The level of success of the application of recombinant DNA techniques to vaccine production in social, economic, or financial terms, however, still remains to be seen. This chapter aims to point out some of the scientific avenues that are being actively pursued.

A. What Are Recombinant DNA Techniques?

Recombinant DNA techniques are so called because they enable DNA molecules to be recombined *in vitro*. The procedures rely on the fundamental observation that sequence-specific restriction enzymes cut DNA from virtually any source to generate fragments with termini that can be rejoined. Cutting DNA from different sources with the same enzyme allows the recombination of DNA from widely diverse organisms. The techniques are also referred to as *gene cloning* because when a heterogeneous set of DNA fragments generated by restriction enzyme digestion are inserted into an autonomously replicating vector molecule (usually a plasmid or a virus containing a selectable marker) and transferred into a host (either prokaryotic or eukaryotic) by transformation, the process gives rise to discrete colonies or clones, each containing a unique piece of DNA. Provided a selection or screening procedure is available, a plasmid containing a particular DNA fragment can be isolated from the "library" of colonies, and grown in large amounts and subsequently analysed. Several different plasmid and phage vector systems have been derived for cloning DNAs of different sizes in *Escherichia coli* (see Old and Primrose, 1981). For isolating complete eukaryotic genes, some of which are several kilobases (kb) long owing to the introns interrupting the coding regions, vectors based on phage λ are used (Brammar, 1982).

The genomes of several DNA viruses have been cloned in *E. coli* by one or other of these routes, and some of their nucleotide sequences have been obtained. The genes coding for some bacterial and parasite surface antigens and bacterial toxins have also been isolated in this way and sequenced. For viruses with RNA genomes, this kind of direct "shotgun" cloning is not appropriate because RNA is not cleaved by restriction enzymes. Instead, DNA copies of the RNA are made by using reverse transcriptase, and the cDNA (copy DNA) is cloned into plasmid vectors by homopolymer tailing or by using oligonucleotide linkers (see Williams, 1981).

Systems for the expression of cloned genes in *E. coli* have been developed using vectors containing the necessary bacterial sequence elements to ensure that transcription and translation takes place, e.g., a promoter sequence and ribosome binding site. Figure 1 shows the two different strategies used to obtain expression of cloned genes in *E. coli*. The genes are either expressed as fusion proteins where existing bacterial transcription and translation initiation signals are retained in the plasmid, giving rise to a hybrid protein consisting of the "foreign" polypeptide fused to the amino terminal part of a bacterial protein, or as native proteins where the 5′ end of the cloned gene is positioned adjacent to the bacterial promoter driving transcription in the plasmid, giving rise to the foreign protein with an amino terminal methionine residue.*

A variety of cloning and expression vectors have been constructed for industrially important bacteria[†]. Similar expression vectors for *Saccharomyces cerevisiae* and mammalian cells have also been developed. These vectors contain analogous structural elements to those in *E. coli* vectors, i.e. a marker gene to enable selection of cells containing the vector, an origin of DNA replication, a controllable promoter and other transcriptional signals plus suitable restriction sites in which to clone foreign DNA. Promoters from genes

---

*See Harris (1983) for a review of the expression of eukaryotic genes in *E. coli*.

†For example Streptomyces (Chater *et al.*, 1982) and *Bacillus subtilis* (Kreft and Hughes, 1982).

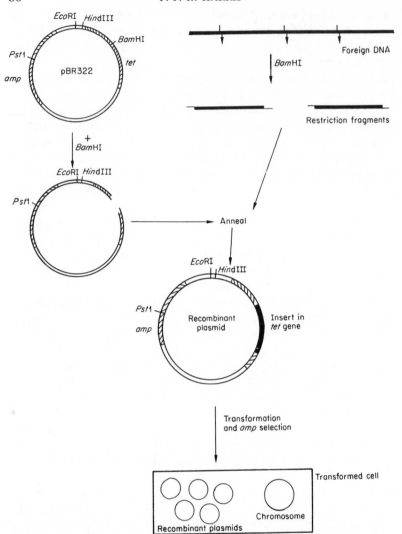

Fig. 1. A simple cloning experiment. A heterogeneous set of DNA fragments generated by digestion of DNA with the restriction enzyme *Bam*H1 are ligated to the *E. coli* plasmid vector pBR322 digested with the same enzyme. Bacteria containing recombinant plasmids are selected on agar plates containing ampicillin, since the tetracycline resistance gene (*tet*) is inactivated by insertion of DNA into the *Bam*H1 site, whereas the ampicillin resistance gene (*amp*) is not affected. The sites of action of the other restriction enzymes *Pst*1, *Eco*RI, and *Hin*dIII are also shown.

involved in glycolysis are often used to initiate transcription in yeast expression plasmids because these enzymes are usually expressed to a high level (e.g., phosphoglycerate kinase), coupled to an origin of replication derived from the 2μ endogenous yeast plasmid (Beggs, 1981; Hinnen and Meyhack, 1982; Hollenberg, 1982). The mammalian cell vectors are largely based on viruses that infect mammalian cells, e.g., SV40 or bovine papilloma virus (BPV). Depending on what sort of vector is used, exogenous DNA can be maintained episomally or integrated into the chromosome of the cell (Rigby, 1982, 1983). In most cases these mammalian cell vectors contain in addition, an *E. coli* origin of replication and selectable marker so that the recombinants can be made and characterised and amplified in *E. coli* before being transferred to the host organism.

B. Existing Vaccines

It is hardly appropriate to discuss novel approaches to vaccines using gene manipulation without some appreciation of the existing technology, especially as some of these vaccines are the very ones with which recombinant DNA derived products will have to compete. There are two types of vaccine in use today, killed or live (attenuated). These two categories can be further subdivided into bacterial or virus vaccines and into whole organism or subunit (split) vaccines (Table I).

There is a general consensus that the immunity conferred by live vaccines is superior to that induced by inactivated vaccines. Many live vaccines give an efficient long-lasting immune response after one "dose", whereas inactivated vaccines usually have to be given repeatedly under controlled conditions. However, the fact that both live attenuated (Sabin) and inactivated (Salk) poliovirus vaccines can be equally effective under certain conditions is a good illustration of the utility of both types of vaccine. Table I is a list of the types of vaccine presently in use and provides some examples for each type, although it is not an exhaustive catalogue of currently available vaccines. In general, there are fewer bacterial vaccines than virus vaccines and many of the latter are for veterinary use.

It is interesting that recombinant DNA techniques have been applied to most of these different vaccine types (Table II). Subunit

TABLE I Types of Existing Vaccine[a]

Inactivated (killed) vaccines	
Whole organisms	
Bacteria	B. pertussis (whooping cough); S. typhosa, S. paratyphi (typhoid); V. cholera (cholera); B. abortus (brucellosis); B. anthracis (anthrax)
Viruses	Rabies, influenza, polio (Salk vaccine) foot-and-mouth disease, animal parvoviruses
Subunit vaccines	
Formalin-fixed toxin (toxoid)	C. tetani (tetanus); C. diphtheriae (diphtheria)
"Split" components	Hepatitis B surface antigen; influenza HA and NM; adenovirus
Live vaccines	
Bacteria	M. tuberculosis (BCG); B. abortus (brucellosis)
Viruses	
Naturally occurring	Vaccinia, Turkey herpes (Marek's disease); rubella (German measles), Newcastle disease, infectious bronchitis
"Adapted"	Mumps, measles, polio (Sabin), yellow fever
"Reassorted"	Influenza, rotavirus (experimental)

[a]See Norrby (1983); Beale and Harris (1979).

vaccines for both bacterial and virus antigens are being prepared by expression of the relevant surface immunogens in *E. coli* or other hosts. Protein sequence information is being derived from nucleotide sequence data obtained from cloned genes, enabling peptides of defined amino acid sequence to be made for use as immunogens (Lerner, 1983), and novel live recombinant viruses are being constructed.

II. EXPRESSION OF IMMUNOGENS IN *E. COLI*

A. Expression of Bacterial Antigens

Despite the fact that some of the earliest cloned genes expressed in *E. coli* were viral antigens, the first commercial vaccine prepared

TABLE II Recombinant DNA Approaches to Vaccines

Subunit vaccines
  1. Expression of immunogenic polypeptides in genetically engineered prokaryotic
     or eukaryotic hosts
  2. Carrier-conjugated synthetic peptides where amino acid sequences have been
     derived from cloned DNA
Live vaccines
  1. Genetic reassortment *in vivo,* e.g., between the RNAs of different influenza
     viruses
  2. Modification of DNA by *in vitro* mutation, e.g., the modification of cloned
     poliovirus infectious DNA
  3. Modification of virus DNA *in vitro* using restriction enzymes, e.g.,
     adenoviruses, herpesviruses
  4. Antigens cloned in vaccinia virus, e.g., hepatitis B surface antigen, influenza
     HA

---

by this route is against a bacterial pilus antigen. Pathogenic forms of enteric bacteria possess surface proteinaceous fimbriae or pili that enable them to adhere to and colonise cell membranes. The genes coding for the pilus antigens of enterotoxigenic *E. coli* (e.g., K88, K99, CFA/1, and CFA/2) have been cloned and expressed in nonpathogenic *E. coli* (e.g., K12) to produce large amounts of fimbrial protein free from enterotoxin contamination, which has been formulated into a vaccine. A similar approach is being used for the gonococcal pilus antigen. An alternative has been to prepare nontoxigenic K88 bacteria by *in vitro* modification of the toxin genes present on a resident plasmid. This approach is also being applied to *Vibrio cholera.* Nontoxigenic live *V. cholera* strains have been proposed as alternative vaccines to the killed vaccines presently in use because these are relatively ineffective and induce only a short-lived immunity. Whether these kinds of methods will be successful for other bacteria (e.g., *B. pertussis*), where the precise contribution of pilus antigens, outer membrane proteins, and lipopolysacharrides to immunogenicity has not been determined, is very much an open question.

B. Expression of Virus Glycoproteins

One of the first virus antigens to be expressed in *E. coli* with the intention of making a subunit vaccine was the haemagglutinin (HA) of fowl plague influenza virus. This protein is responsible for eliciting the formation of neutralising antibody during influenza infection, although antibodies to the neuraminidase (NM, the other virus envelope protein) are thought to play a role in limiting virus spread. Conventional subunit vaccines against influenza based on these two antigens are available but are not without problems. The most notable is the frequency with which new strains of the virus arise. This is caused by both antigenic drift where point mutations occur in the surface proteins and antigenic shift where one or other of the genes encoding surface proteins is replaced by a similar gene acquired from an animal strain (eg., subtypes H_1, H_2, and H_3). The eight segments of single stranded (ss) RNA that make up the genome of influenza virus facilitates this kind of genetic reassortment.*

A DNA copy of the fowl plague virus HA gene (segment 4 of the RNA) has been cloned into an *E. coli* expression vector downstream of a *trp* promoter (the promoter from the tryptophan operon of *E. coli*), so that a complete HA polypeptide was synthesised (Emtage *et al.*, 1980). Immunoreactive protein was detected in induced cultures of plasmid bearing bacteria (i.e., in the absence of tryptophan), but the levels of expression were considerably lower than expected. More recently, higher levels of expression of a human influenza HA have been reported in *E. coli*. In these studies, the complete HA and two N-terminal truncated derivatives were produced as fusion proteins to part of the *trpE* protein (the first gene in the *trp* operon). These HA derivatives elicited antibodies that recognised native HA, but they were clearly not identical to antibodies elicited by native HA. Furthermore, no protection studies were done (Davis *et al.*, 1983).

Essentially the same strategy has been used to express other virus glycoproteins in *E. coli* with similar results (Table III). The first efforts to express hepatitis B surface antigen (HBsAg) in microorganisms, for example, were done in *E. coli* (Table III), and parts of the spike protein (the G or glycoprotein) of rabies virus have also been made this way. Vaccines to rabies virus, one of the first human diseases for which a systematically developed vaccine was prepared, are currently made by inactivating virus grown in tissue culture. This is an inefficient procedure, owing to poor growth of the virus in cell culture, so there is considerable interest in alterna-

*See Lamb and Choppin (1983) for a review of influenza virus structure and replication.

tive sources of antigen. Unfortunately, the NH_2 and COOH terminal hydrophobic regions of the rabies G protein are toxic to *E. coli* cells, and reasonably high levels of expression can only be obtained if these sequences are removed (Yelverton *et al.*, 1983). This is particularly unfortunate for the rabies G protein because the COOH terminal hydrophobic domain is required for efficient production of virus neutralising antibodies in immunised animals (Wunner *et al.*, 1983). These studies actually highlight several of the problems that seem to be inherent in the expression of eukaryotic proteins in *E. coli* (see Harris, 1983). Apart from the toxic effects of hydrophobic domains, proteins that are normally glycosylated remain free from carbohydrate when synthesised in *E. coli;* some carbohydrate moieties may be important for immunogenicity. Furthermore, most eukaryotic proteins (even truncated fusion proteins) are insoluble in *E. coli*, forming inclusion bodies that require the use of powerful protein denaturants such as guanidine hydrochloride to solubilise them. This treatment may again drastically affect immunogenicity. With the promising development of expression systems for eukaryotic cells (see Section IV), it seems unlikely that *E. coli* will be the microorganism of choice for producing many subunit antigens.

C. Expression of FMDV VP1

The possible exception to this is the expression of nonglycosylated and less hydrophobic virus proteins. An example of an immunogen of this kind is the capsid virus protein VP1 of foot-and-mouth disease virus (FMDV). Foot-and-mouth disease is controlled by vaccination in the parts of the world where it is enzootic, although an isolation and slaughter policy is maintained elsewhere. The vaccines are produced by inactivation of virus grown on a large scale in BHK cells or bovine tongue epithelium. The vaccines are generally effective when administered properly but are not without problems. For example, the virus particles, even when inactivated, are unstable below pH 7 and are heat sensitive. The vaccine problem is further compounded by the fact that there are seven serotypes of FMDV (classified on the basis of cross protection immunity) and many subtypes within each virus serotype; differences between subtypes cause, in some instances, a loss of cross-protection. There

TABLE III   Expression of Virus Immunogens in Prokaryotic and Eukaryotic Cells

Antigen	Cell type	Construction	Comment	Reference
FMDV VP1	E. coli	trp LE' fusion	High expression levels	See Harris, 1983
	B. subtilis	Erythromycin resistance gene fusion	Low level of synthesis	See Harris, 1983
Polio virus VP1	E. coli	β-Lactamase fusion	Low level of synthesis	Van der Werf et al., 1983
Vesicular stomatitis virus (VSV) G protein	E. coli	trp driven trp E fusion	High levels of expression of G protein only if hydrophobic regions removed	See Harris, 1983
Rabies virus G protein	E. coli	trp driven native protein and β lactamase fusion	See VSV G protein	Yelverton et al., 1983
Influenza HA	E. coli	trp driven fusions	Only hydrophobic region minus truncated proteins expressed to high level.	See Harris, 1983; Davis et al., 1983
	Monkey cells	SV40 early and late gene replacement vectors	Cell surface expression of intact HA, no cleavage to HA1 & HA2. "Anchor" minus HA secreted.	Sveda et al., 1982; Gething and Sambrook, 1981, 1982
	Rabbits	Vaccinia recombinant	Antibody raised in vaccinated animals	Panicali et al., 1983

Protein	Host	Vector/method	Comments	References
HBsAg	*E. coli*	Various fusions, some truncated derivatives	Generally low levels of expression owing to hydrophobic regions	See Harris *et al.*, 1983; Fujisawa *et al.*, 1983
	Yeast	Different yeast promoters directing expression of native HBsAg from 2μ-based plasmids	Monomer and 22-nm particles of HBsAg formed	Valenzuela *et al.*, 1982; Hitzeman *et al.*, 1983; Miyanohara *et al.*, 1983
	Mouse cells	Co-transfection with the DHFR (dihydrofolate reductase) gene	Continuous cell line produced by methotrexate selection; 22-nm particles produced	Christman *et al.*, 1982
	Mouse cells	BPV vectors	Transformed cell lines; 22-nm particles produced	Stenlund *et al.*, 1983; Wang *et al.*, 1983.
	Monkey cells	SV40 late gene replacement vector	Infected cells make 22-nm particles	Moriarty *et al.*, 1981
	Rabbits, chimpanzees	Vaccinia recombinants	Rabbits make neutralising antibody; chimpanzees are protected from hepatitis B	Smith *et al.*, 1983
HSV glycoprotein D	*E. coli*	*lac* promoter, λ phage gene fusion protein	Only reasonably high expression levels if large fusion made or hydrophobic domains removed.	Watson *et al.*, 1982

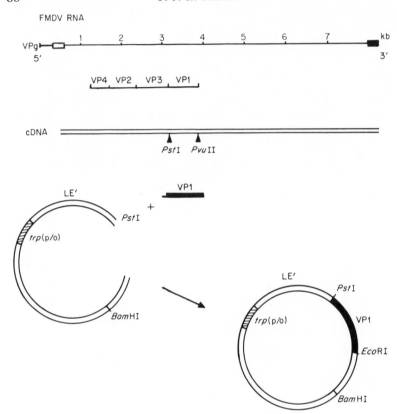

Fig. 2.   Construction of the *E. coli* expression vector for the synthesis of FMDV VP1 as a fusion protein with *trp* LE'. FMDV contains an ss RNA molecule of 8 kb with a poly(A) tract (■) at the 3' end and a poly(C) tract (□) near the 5' end of the RNA close to the genome-linked protein (VPg) at the 5' end. cDNA covering the region of the RNA coding for the structural proteins (VP4, 2, 3, 1) of the virus was synthesised and cloned. The VP1 gene was cut out of the DNA by cleavage with the restriction enzymes *Pst*1 and *Pvu*II and inserted into a fusion vector containing the *trp* promoter operator (p/o) driving transription of the LE' protein to yield a vector expressing the trp LE'-VP1 fusion protein. (Derived from Kleid *et al.*, 1981.)

is also the potential (and actual) problem of insufficient inactivation of vaccine virus, leading to infection of vaccinated animals.

Of the four structural proteins of the virus, it is VP1 that contains the major neutralising epitopes. This was originally suggested by the observation that trypsin treatment of intact virus particles, which specifically cleaved VP1, also reduced the infectivity and immunogenicity of the particles. Moreover, VP1 isolated from virus particles raises neutralising antibodies (see Bittle *et al.*, 1982 for references). Most of the 8 kb ss RNA genome of FMDV has now been cloned, including the region coding for the structural proteins, and vectors have been constructed for the expression of VP1 in *E. coli*. Kleid *et al.* (1981) made a vector containing the *trp* promoter, designed to direct the synthesis of VP1 linked to a hybrid protein consisting of the NH_2-terminus of the trp leader peptide fused to the last one-third of the *trp* E protein (Fig. 2). This *trp* LE' fragment is a particularly useful protein for fusions because it is insoluble and resistant to proteolysis. Relatively large amounts of the *trp* LE' VP1 fusion protein (170 mg from 800 ml of culture or about 17% of total cell protein) were obtained in the pellet from a detergent lysate of bacteria. After purification by gel electrophoresis, the protein was mixed with adjuvant and used to vaccinate both swine and cattle. As might be expected, the fusion protein was no better as an immunogen than VP1 isolated from virus particles, but it did elicit the formation of reasonably high levels of neutralising antibody and some vaccinated animals were protected from disease on challenge. The high level of expression of the fusion protein should now enable studies of antigen presentation and of the effect of adjuvants on the immunogenicity of this protein made this way to be assessed.

III. EXPRESSION OF VIRUS GLYCOPROTEINS IN YEAST

Hepatitis B Surface Antigen

The lack of success of expressing complete virus glycoproteins in *E. coli* automatically led to an examination of expression in other organisms fermentable on a large scale. For this reason and because vectors were becoming available, yeast (*Saccharomyces cerevisiae*) was the organism of choice. Compared to *E. coli*, relatively few ''foreign'' genes have been expressed in yeast; of those that have, one of the most well expressed is HBsAg, a protein that is not well expressed in *E. coli* (see Section II).

Most of the newer hepatitis B virus (HBV) vaccines currently in use are based on 22-nm lipoprotein particles made up of the surface antigen. These particles, found in the plasma of asymptomatic carriers of the disease, are purified extensively and then formulated into vaccines (Zuckerman, 1982). Although the vaccine is efficacious and protects individuals against hepatitis B, the vaccine is expensive owing to the high degree of purification necessary to ensure complete removal of infective virus and host material and to the safety testing that has to be done in chimpanzees.

The DNA of three of the four subtypes of hepatitis B virus has now been cloned, and the sequences of the surface antigens have been compared (Fujiyama *et al.*, 1983). The surface antigen has a molecular weight of about 23,00 and exists in both unglycosylated and glycosylated forms (MW 26,000–29,000).

The engineering of HBsAg for expression in yeast has been reported by at least three groups (Valenzuela *et al.*, 1982, Hitzeman *et al.*, 1983; Miyanohara *et al.*, 1983), each using a different yeast promoter to drive transcription across the HBsAg gene (Fig. 3). Not only was HBsAg produced in yeast from these plasmid constructions, but 22-nm particles were formed, which apparently had the same physicochemical properties as natural 22-nm particles and induced comparable levels of HBsAg antibodies in mice (Fig. 4). However, higher levels of monomer HBsAg were formed than of

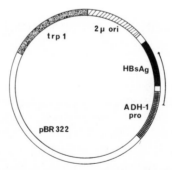

Fig. 3.   Plasmid expression vector for the synthesis of hepatitis B surface antigen (HBsAg) in yeast. The plasmid consists of an origin of replication from the 2μ plasmid (2μ ori) linked to a selection marker (*trp* 1) and sequences from the *E. coli* plasmid pBR322. Transcription of the HBsAg gene is driven by the alcohol dehydrogenase gene promotor (ADH-1). (Adapted from Valenzuela *et al.*, 1982.)

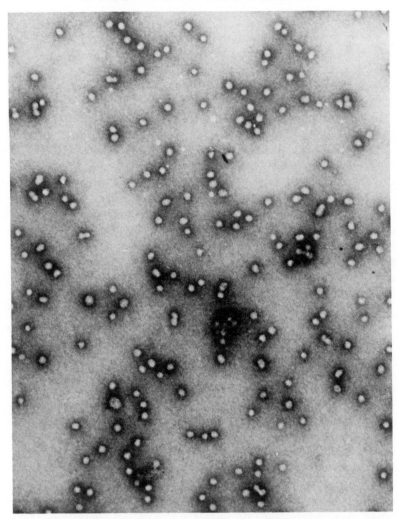

Fig. 4   Electron micrograph of 22-nm HBsAg particles made in yeast cells. Particles were purified by immunoaffinity chromatography and negatively stained with 2% phosphotungstic acid. (Photograph by courtesy of Dr. P. Valenzuela, Chiron Corp.)

the 22-nm particle. Because it has been shown that protein micelles of HBsAg, produced by detergent treatment, elicit a more vigorous immune response in mice than 22-nm particles, it is possible that monomer-based vaccines could be prepared from material made in yeast (Zuckerman, 1982). Recently, yeast derived HBsAg has been shown to induce protective antibodies in chimpanzees (K. Murray, personal communication).

IV. EXPRESSION OF VIRUS GLYCOPROTEINS IN HIGHER EUKARYOTIC CELLS

A. Hepatitis B Surface Antigen

Most of the molecules of HBsAg formed in yeast are not glycosylated or are glycosylated improperly (Valenzuela *et al.*, 1982). Consequently, there has been considerable interest in expressing HBsAg in higher eukaryotic cells where full glycosylation should occur. Several different approaches have been used to do this, using either co-transfection of cells with cloned virus DNA or by means of eukaryotic virus vectors. One of the viruses that has been extensively used for this purpose is the simian virus SV40. The virus contains a small circular DNA molecule. During infection, this DNA is transcribed into mRNA (which is then translated into virus-specific proteins) in two phases. The "early" genes, which code for the nonstructural proteins, e.g., large T and small t antigens, are transcribed before DNA replication and the "late" genes, which code for virus structural proteins, are expressed after DNA replication. Using an SV40 late gene replacement vector* (where the late genes of the virus were replaced with HBsAg DNA and the recombinant virus DNA propagated in the presence of an SV40 early gene mutant to provide late gene functions), Moriarty *et al.*, (1981) demonstrated the synthesis of HBsAg in infected monkey kidney cells. Some of the protein was found in the medium in the form of 22-nm particles. These had the same glycosylation patterns and antigenic properties as 22-nm particles isolated from infected plasma or from a continuously producing hepatoma cell line. These SV40 vectors however, are infective and do not lead to the establishment of cell lines.

Establishing cell lines producing HBsAg (rather than infection) can be done by transfection of cells with HBV DNA under certain conditions or by using other recombinant virus vectors. For example, co-transfection of cells with HBV DNA and a dihydrofolate

*See Fig. 6 for the structure of an SV40 late gene replacement vector.

reductase gene (DHFR) has led to the establishment of a methotrexate resistant cell line that produces HBsAg because cells that have taken up the DHFR gene and are resistant to methotrexate also take up the HBV DNA. Under increased methotrexate selection, the chromosomally integrated viral DNA sequences are amplified along with the DHFR gene, which provides more enzyme to overcome the effect of the methotrexate; considerable amounts of HBsAg accumulate in the medium in the form of 22-nm particles (Christman *et al.*, 1982). The surface antigen gene has also been introduced into vectors based on bovine papilloma virus (BPV). These vectors are in many respects the mouse cell equivalents of prokaryotic plasmid vectors (Fig. 5) (Wang *et al.*, 1983; Stenlund *et al.*, 1983). As with the co-transfected cells, the BPV/HBsAg transformed cell lines make 22-nm particles identical to those present in carrier serum. The amounts of HBsAg produced in the two types of recombinant cell lines are similar ($50–200$ ng/10^6 cells), a good deal higher than those obtained from hepatoma cell lines. Further "fine tuning" of the expression vectors (e.g., by including a stronger promoter and a relevant enhancer sequence) may well increase the amount of HBsAg that can be synthesised. Nevertheless, it has yet to be shown that HBsAg particles produced in transformed cell lines can protect chimpanzees from infection, although specific antibodies are apparently produced in guinea pigs (Wang

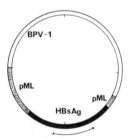

Fig. 5. Structure of a bovine papilloma virus (BPV)-based vector for the expression of HBsAg in mouse cells. In this construction transcription occurs from the HBsAg promoter upstream of the gene. The BPV DNA provides an origin of DNA replication and transforms cells into foci providing a method of selection. pML is a derivative of the *E. coli* plasmid pBR322 included to allow construction and characterisation of the plasmid in *E. coli* before transformation of the mouse cells. (Derived from Stenlund *et al.*, 1983.)

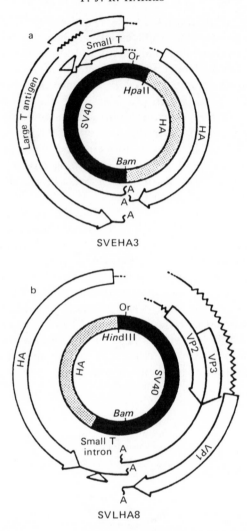

Fig. 6. SV40-HA recombinants designed to express influenza haemagglutinin in monkey cells. The shaded circles represent the DNA of the recombinant viruses (□ = HA; ■ = SV40 DNA). Untranslated portions of mRNA are shown as solid lines with dots indicating 5′ ends, zigzag lines showing segments spliced out of the transcripts, and wavy lines the poly(A) tails at the 3′ end of the DNA. Protein coding regions are indicated by blocked arrows. (a) SVE HA3 is the late gene replacement vector retaining the SV40 early gene transcription unit (left-hand side of the plasmid) with the influenza

et al., 1983). If chimpanzees are protected, then it is a question of whether eukaryotic cell expression of HBsAg will compete in economic terms with the yeast system, e.g., in terms of costs of tissue culture medium compared to feedstock or other downstream processing considerations. It will also be necessary to confirm the nature of the immune response to particles derived from each source.

B. Influenza HA

The only other virus immunogen that has been expressed in eukaryotic cells in a similar way is the influenza HA. In an elegant series of experiments, monkey cells were infected with both SV40 late and early gene replacement vectors (Fig. 6; Gething and Sambrook, 1981, 1982). The late gene vectors were propagated in a similar way to the HBsAg late gene replacement vectors. The early gene replacement vectors were propagated in COS-1 cells, which endogenously express SV40 large T antigen and can thus by complementation help the vector and give rise to a fully recombinant virus stock (i.e., not contaminated with helper virus). Cells infected with either type of recombinant synthesise HA. About 80 μg of protein is produced per dish of cells infected with the late vector recombinant. As with other similar studies (Sveda and Lai, 1981), the HA produced was glycosylated (but not cleaved to HA1 and HA2) and was located at the cell surface. Similar vectors containing deleted derivatives of the HA gene (missing either the NH$_2$ terminal hydrophobic signal or the COOH terminal anchor domain) have also been constructed (Sveda *et al.*, 1982, Gething and Sambrook, 1982). HA lacking the signal is only produced at low levels in infected cells, whereas HA minus the anchor is glycosylated and secreted into the medium. These experiments not only yield interesting information about the structure and synthesis of membrane proteins, but they illustrate what "may become a general method for obtaining with ease large quantities of purified eukary-

---

HA gene replacing the late genes. (b) SVL HA8 is the early gene replacement vector where the late SV40 gene transcription unit is retained (right-hand side of the plasmid) the early gene region being replaced by the influenza HA gene. [Reprinted by permission from Gething and Sambrook (1981), *Nature (London)* 293, 620-625. Copyright 1981 MacMillan Journals Ltd.]

yotic membrane antigens for experimental analysis or vaccine production'' (Gething and Sambrook, 1982). Although this may be true for viruses that are not easy to grow to high titres (e.g., rabies virus), one wonders whether it will be true for other viruses that do grow to high titres and with several glycoprotein antigens, e.g., some herpes viruses.

Nevertheless, the stage has been set for the construction of vectors containing a number of different virus glycoprotein genes and for their insertion into eukaryotic cells to make transformed lines. The immunogenic properties of the continually synthesised polypeptides can then be analysed in detail. So far, the results are certainly more encouraging than those obtained by expression of these virus genes in *E. coli.*

V. USE OF SYNTHETIC PEPTIDES AS IMMUNOGENS

The groundwork for using short synthetic peptides as immunogens was laid when it was found that a hexapeptide from the COOH terminus of tobacco mosaic virus coupled to bovine serum albumin (BSA) induced the production of antibodies that could precipitate and neutralise the virus.* In work with MS_2 phage, it was also shown that two synthetic peptides representing parts of the coat protein of the virus produced antibody that under certain circumstances would bind to the virus.

The full potential of immunization with synthetic peptides, however, could not be realised until recombinant DNA techniques were developed. Access to cloned genes has enabled the nucleotide sequence of many virus nucleic acids to be obtained from which amino acid sequences have been derived.

The amino acid sequence of HBsAg and influenza HA from several different virus subtypes has been deduced, and the sequence of VP1 for at least three of the seven serotypes of FMDV has been obtained. The availability of these sequences has allowed an examination of the conserved and variable regions in the proteins. In addition, hydrophobicity and hydrophilicity histograms have been derived using computer programmes. In general, it has been found that the hydrophilic (and probably solvent exposed) regions of the

*For detailed reviews of synthetic peptide vaccines, see Arnon *et al.* (1983) and this volume, Chapter 4, Sutcliffe *et al.* (1983), or Lerner (1982, 1983).

proteins tend to be more variable than the hydrophobic domains. This suggests that it is these regions that are involved in the raising of neutralising antibodies. To test this reasoning, peptides have been synthesised covering regions of HBsAg, influenza HA, and FMDV VP1, and their immunogenicity analysed.

A. HBsAg Peptides

Immunochemically, HBsAg consists of group specific determinants (a) and two subtype specific determinants (d/y and w/r) (Tiollais *et al.*, 1981). Computer predictions from amino acid sequences indicate that the molecule is composed of three hydrophobic and two hydrophilic regions. Comparative sequence analysis of HBsAg from different subtypes shows that these hydrophilic regions are more variable than the hydrophobic ones, suggesting that the subtype specificity domains lie in the hydrophilic regions (Fujiyama *et al.*, 1983). Peptides from one of the hydrophilic regions (amino acids 109–150) synthesised by at least five different groups have been shown to raise HBsAg specific antibodies in mice or rabbits when coupled to carrier proteins (see Arnon *et al.*, 1983). The antisera raised by different peptides has given some direct evidence of where subtype and group specific determinants lie on HBsAg, but in only one study has any protection data been reported. Here a peptide consisting of amino acids 110–137 of the y subtype coupled to keyhole limpet haemocyanin (KLH) was used to immunise three chimpanzees (1 mg peptide/0.5 ml dose intramuscularly, each with a different adjuvant, two doses, 5 weeks apart). Primary and secondary responses were found in all three animals, but the responses were transient. Indeed, even after repeated vaccination stable anti-HBsAg failed to be maintained in the animals, and only one chimpanzee was protected against subsequent inoculation with hepatitis B virus (Gerin *et al.*, 1983). On this evidence, then, there is clearly some way to go yet before synthetic peptides can be considered as vaccines for hepatitis B.

B. FMDV VP1 Peptides

Much more convincing data has been presented for the foot-and-mouth disease virus immunogenic capsid protein VP1. By using enzymatic and chemical cleavage methods, it had been shown that two C terminal regions of the protein were responsible for inducing neutralising antibody (Strohmaier *et al.,* 1982). A comparison of the nucleotide sequences of this region of several serotypes of FMDV has indicated that there are two variable regions in the COOH terminal part of VPl; these correspond to the major immunogenic sites found from the protein studies (Makoff *et al.,* 1982). On the basis of these results, several peptides have been synthesised to regions of VPl, including peptides spanning the variable regions from amino acid 141–160 and 200–213. Not only do these peptides raise high levels of neutralising antibody in rabbits when coupled to KLH, but inoculations of guinea pigs with the conjugates leads to some protection of the animals from infection on subsequent challenge with homologous virus (Bittle *et al.,* 1982; Pfaff *et al.,* 1982). The amount of neutralising antibody raised by a single inoculation of the 141–160 conjugate was less than 10% of that obtained from a single inoculation of an equal weight of inactivated virus, where VPl is constrained in the virus particle, but much greater than that obtained by inoculation with isolated VPl or the *trp* LE[1] VPl fusion protein made in *E. coli.* Furthermore, the synthetic peptides mimic the subtype specificity of the virus, i.e., the antibody synthesised in response to a 141–160 peptide with the sequence of type A10 virus neutralises homologous virus better than another type A virus and vice versa (Clarke *et al.,* 1983). Unfortunately, as yet, no challenge studies have been reported for cattle immunised with synthetic FMDV peptides, although peptide 141–160 elicits a neutralising antibody response in cattle and pigs, which should be sufficient for protection against disease (Bittle *et al.,* 1982).

It is not inconceivable that peptide vaccines could be used for FMDV because they eliminate several of the problems with the current inactivated vaccines. In particular, if subtype specificity is controlled by variation in only one or two amino acids in VPl, it should be relatively straightforward to identify virus variants in the field simply by growing the virus and obtaining the nucleotide sequence across this part of the VP1 gene. The relevant peptide can then be synthesised, formulated, and used as a vaccine in the geographical area from which the virus was isolated. Nevertheless, in view of the fact that the current vaccines are reasonably efficient, it seems more likely that the FMDV model will form a paradigm for other viruses for which no vaccine is available. One that comes immediately to mind is hepatitis A, a disease also caused by a picornavirus. Hepatitis A virus RNA is now being cloned and sequenced by several groups, no doubt with this thought in mind.

C. Influenza HA Peptides

Comparative nucleotide sequence data are also available for influenza HA, and immunogenic peptides have also been synthesised for this molecule. In this case, however, there was no need for a computer prediction of hydrophilic (surface) or hydrophobic regions to indicate which peptides to synthesise, because the three dimensional structure of influenza HA had been established by X-ray crystallography (Wiley *et al.*, 1981). The HA molecule on the virus particle is a trimeric molecule consisting of three copies of HA1 and HA2. A single monomer (Fig. 7) looks like an elongated cylinder with a stem comprised mainly of HA2 and a globular head consisting entirely of HA1 residues.* Amino acid sequences derived from the nucleotide sequence of various cloned HA genes, of both natural subtype H3 variants and of H3 variants selected by monoclonal antibodies, have indicated that there are four major antigenic determinants on the HA, mostly located on the globular head of the molecule. Although peptides have been made covering much of the surface of the HA1 molecule (Green *et al.*, 1982) and have been shown to raise specific HA antibodies, most of these sera do not neutralise the virus. However, immunisations with several combinations of peptides from HA1 apparently protect mice from death caused by mouse-adapted influenza virus (Sutcliffe *et al.*, 1983).

Peptides made to a conserved region near the NH$_2$ terminus of HA2 also seem to raise antibodies that neutralise virus in a tissue culture assay and in a subtype independent way (Sutcliffe *et al.*, 1983; Arnon *et al.*, 1983). More work is needed to see if these peptides or others similar to them can protect animals from disease caused by one or several of the virus subtypes.

*See Lamb and Choppin (1983) for a review of influenza virus structure and replication.

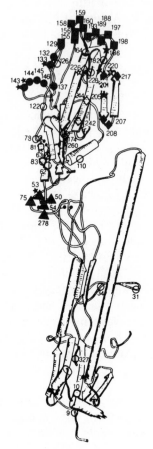

Fig. 7.   Schematic drawing of a monomer of influenza (A/Aichi/68) haemagglutinin. Cylinders represent α helices; flat twisted arrows, β chains; and small filled lollipops, disulphide bridges. The globular head of the molecule consists of HA1 attached to HA2 which predominantly makes up the elongated stem. Amino acid substitutions observed between 1968–1979 are marked and grouped into five regions (○, ●, ▲, ◆, ■). Stars indicate the positions of amino acid substitutions observed in HAs of antigenic variants selected using monoclonal antibodies. (Photograph by courtesy of Dr. John Skehel; see Wiley *et al.*, 1981; see also Lamb and Choppin, 1983 for further detail.)

D. Poliovirus Peptides

Monoclonal antibodies have also been used to try to identify the antigenic determinant(s) involved in producing neutralising antibody to poliovirus. This virus is yet another one belonging to the picornavirus family and exists in three serotypes (polio 1, polio 2, polio 3). Naturally occurring mutant polio type 3 viruses have been selected by resistance to neutralisation by a panel of monoclonal antibodies and the mutations screened and located in the RNA genome by RNase T_1 fingerprinting. A specific oligonucleotide was found to be absent from the mutants, and nucleotide sequencing revealed that this oligonucleotide was derived from a region about 300 nucleotides into the poliovirus VP1 gene (Minor *et al.*, 1983). Further nucleotide sequencing in this region of the RNA (for representatives of 16 groups of mutant viruses) shows that most of the mutations conferring resistance to neutralisation are confined to an eight amino acid stretch of VP1 coded for by residues 277–300 (Evans *et al.*, 1983). This implies that these amino acids represent the major epitope for neutralisation on the virus. Also as might be expected, there is low overall homology between this sequence in type 3 virus and the sequence in this part of VP1 from polio type 1. A peptide covering this region of VP1 of poliovirus type 1 raises neutralising antibodies in rabbits when conjugated to BSA as a carrier. Other peptides from VP1 do not raise neutralising antibodies but prime rabbits to produce virus neutralising antibodies after inoculation with intact virus (Emini *et al.*, 1983). The idea of the peptide priming of an immune response is a new tactic in the strategy of peptide immunogens; it will be interesting to see whether priming with peptides will give any measure of protection against naturally acquired infection.

VI. RECOMBINANT LIVE VACCINES

Most of this chapter has been concerned with the production of subunit vaccines, which come under the heading of inactivated vaccines (Table I). Three categories of live vaccines are in use today (Table I; see Norrby, 1983). Vaccination with cowpox virus (vaccinia), which heralded the whole concept of immunisation, represents an example of the use of infection with a virus that is closely related to a pathogen (in this case smallpox, variola virus) but that is relatively apathogenic, to produce cross-reactive and protective neutralising antibodies. Other more recent examples are available as well, e.g., the control of Marek's disease of chickens with turkey herpesvirus.

More often however, live attenuated virus vaccines have been made by adaptation of virulent viruses to unnatural host cells. Two of the older more successful examples are the 17D strain of yellow fever virus, attenuated by growth in chick embryo cells and the Sabin poliovirus strains, attenuated by growth in monkey kidney cells. Live attenuated measles, rubella (german measles), and mumps vaccines have been produced in the same way. There have been attempts to use temperature-sensitive mutants of respiratory syncytial virus (a paramyxovirus-like virus and a cause of serious lower respiratory tract infection in young children) as an attenuated virus vaccine, but success has been limited. For viruses with segmented genomes (e.g., the myxoviruses-influenza) the technique of genetic reassortment has been used to generate attenuated viruses. This has been done by recombining (that is reassorting) the RNA of viruses from different sources (e.g., avian influenza viruses and mutant human influenza viruses), followed by selection of a virus with the desired attenuated properties and right surface protein subtype specificity. The lack of genetic stability of influenza virus recombinants made this way and the problems of antigenic drift make this a difficult task. It is possible that more success will be met with the reoviruses or the rotaviruses, which have segmented double-stranded (ds) RNA genomes.

A. *In Vitro* Mutagenesis

A much more defined approach to attenuation should now be possible by using recombinant DNA techniques, specifically *in vitro* site directed mutagenesis. This technique provides a unique method of introducing point mutations (or deletions) into any piece of cloned DNA in any predetermined position. The method arose from studies with the ss DNA phage ϕX174 but it has mostly been used with DNA cloned into the ss DNA phage M13. This is convenient because cloned genes are often transferred from plasmid to

M13 vectors to facilitate nucleotide sequencing by the dideoxy procedure. The basic principle of *in vitro* mutagenesis involves the extension by *E. coli* DNA polymerase of a short oligonucleotide primer annealed to DNA cloned in M13 (Fig. 8). The oligonucleotide is complementary to a region in the cloned DNA apart from a mismatch or a deletion defining the mutation site. Closed circular double-stranded DNA molecules are formed by ligation of the extended molecules using DNA ligase and these are purified and used to transform competent *E. coli*.

Phage containing mutant sequences are distinguished by various screening procedures (Zoller and Smith, 1982) and the mutant DNA used to replace the normal sequence in the plasmid from which it was derived. It is obvious that this technique now makes it possible to alter cloned DNA at will. The difficulty as far as virulence and attenuation is concerned is knowing which sequences to change. There has been some progress towards analysing the molecular differences between attenuated and virulent viruses, but it is not clear what the differences mean. For example, there are 57 nucleotide differences between Sabin type 1 poliovirus (LSc 2ab) and Mahoney (its virulent parent virus), 21 of which result in amino acid substitutions, some being clustered at the NH_2 terminus of VP1 (Nomoto *et al.*, 1982). Whether these results mean that the changes in VP1 affect virulence remains to be seen. However, the poliovirus system is particularly interesting because plasmids containing a complete copy of poliovirus RNA (as ds cDNA) produce infectious virus when transfected into HeLa cells (Racaniello and Baltimore, 1981). The way should now be open for making defined mutant polioviruses by introducing directed changes in the cDNA based on information obtained from nucleotide sequence comparisons of other virulent and attenuated polioviruses.

B. Natural Recombinant Viruses

Natural "recombinant" DNA viruses have also been isolated. Adenoviruses, which are causes of epidemic respiratory illness in humans, are icosahedral viruses containing a large double stranded DNA molecule (35 kb). Attenuated vaccines to adenoviruses have been prepared by adapting the viruses to grow in monkey kidney

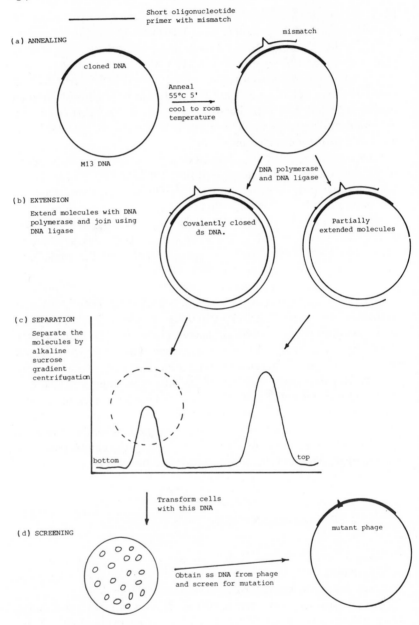

Short oligonucleotide
primer with mismatch

(a) ANNEALING

cloned DNA

mismatch

Anneal
55°C 5'
cool to room
temperature

M13 DNA

DNA polymerase
and DNA ligase

(b) EXTENSION

Extend molecules with DNA
polymerase and join using
DNA ligase

Covalently closed
ds DNA.

Partially
extended molecules

(c) SEPARATION

Separate the
molecules by
alkaline
sucrose
gradient
centrifugation

bottom   top

Transform cells
with this DNA

(d) SCREENING

Obtain ss DNA from phage
and screen for mutation

mutant phage

cells in which they normally undergo an abortive infection. Adenoviruses isolated after extensive passage in the monkey cells were found to be recombinants that had picked up pieces of SV40 DNA from the cells, enabling them to overcome the block to a full infective cycle (Sambrook and Grodzicker, 1980). This finding not only shows the potential of using adenoviruses as vectors for expressing exogenous DNA in tissue culture cells (in the same way as the SV40-based vectors) but it also suggests that it might be possible to use other recombinant viruses constructed *in vitro* directly as attenuated vaccines.

There is considerable potential, for example, for engineering the genome of herpesviruses, which cause a variety of human diseases, for vaccine purposes. The availability of deletion mutants of some herpes simplex viruses (HSV) may help in the construction of attenuated viruses. Nevertheless, the predilection of herpesviruses for causing latent infections, and their oncogenic potential are probably reasons for thinking more in terms of subunit vaccines for these viruses.

C. Vaccinia Recombinants

It is ironic perhaps that most progress towards vaccines of this sort has been made with vaccinia, the archetypal vaccine virus. The feasibility of using vaccinia virus DNA as a vector was established by the cloning of the thymidine kinase (*tk*) gene of HSV. It is not possible to use *in vitro* recombination to insert foreign DNA into the vaccinia genome because it is too large (180 kb). Moreover, isolated virus DNA is not infective; enzymes present in the virus particle are required to initiate transcription of virus DNA in the

---

Fig. 8.   General scheme for oligonucleotide site direct mutagenesis. (a) A short oligonucleotide complementary to a predetermined region in a cloned DNA molecule, apart from a mismatch, is annealed to the DNA cloned in the single-stranded DNA of phage M13. (b) The oligonucleotide is extended using DNA polymerase in the presence of nucleotide precursors and closed circular DNA molecules formed by the action of DNA ligase. (c) These double-stranded molecules are purified from partially extended molecules by alkaline sucrose gradient centrifugation and (d) are used to transform *E. coli*. Mutant phage are selected and mutant DNA recovered. (Adapted from Zoller and Smith, 1982, by permission.)

cytoplasm of infected cells. However, it is possible to insert DNA
into the vaccinia genome by recombination *in vivo*. This was
demonstrated quite clearly by marker rescue experiments where
pieces of vaccinia virus DNA introduced into infected cells were
incorporated into replicating virus DNA and virus particles. A logical extension of this work was to try to insert nonhomologous DNA
into vaccinia virus DNA by transfecting virus-infected cells with
recombinant plasmids that contain foreign DNA sandwiched
between regions of vaccinia DNA. The parts of vaccinia DNA
contained in the plasmid should direct the insertion of the foreign
sequences into the replicating virus DNA (see Fig. 9). This was the
basis of the HSV *tk* experiment. Plasmids containing a piece of
adenovirus DNA inserted within the vaccinia *tk* gene, cloned on a
plasmid, were first transfected into infected cells and *tk* progeny
selected on the basis of resistance to the thymidine analogue
5- bromodeoxyuridine. Analysis of the DNA of these recombinants
showed that the foreign DNA was inserted site specifically into
vaccinia DNA at the *tk* gene locus. The HSV *tk* gene was then
inserted into a similar plasmid, containing a vaccinia virus

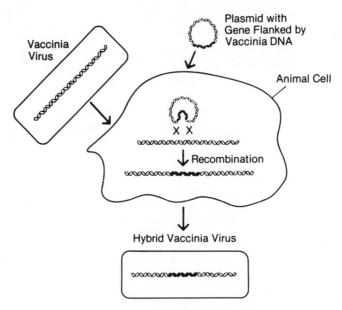

Fig. 9. Diagrammatic representation of the production of recombinant "live"
vaccinia viruses. (By courtesy of Dr. Geoffrey Smith.)

promoter and transfected into tk^- cells infected with a tk^- vaccinia virus. The tk^+ progeny vaccinia virus selected by amethopterin, contain the HSV tk gene inserted site specifically in the DNA, and this provides thymidine kinase to overcome the metabolic block to thymidylate synthesis (Mackett *et al.*, 1982; Panicali and Paoletti, 1982).

This general method has now been used to construct pure vaccinia virus recombinant stocks containing either the influenza HA gene or the HBsAg (Panicali *et al.*, 1983; Smith *et al.*, 1983). Rabbits immunized with the HA recombinants (intravenously) raise high levels of antibody to HA and the serum neutralises virus in a tissue culture assay. However, no protection studies have yet been reported using, for example, vaccinated ferrets. Tissue culture cells infected with the HBsAg recombinant virus synthesise 22-nm particles similar to those obtained from the serum of hepatitis carriers (see Section III) and rabbits vaccinated (intradermally) with purified recombinant virus not only show typical local skin lesions but produce antibodies to HBsAg (Smith *et al.*, 1983). Further experiments with chimpanzees have been done more recently. Despite a low level of specific antibodies following vaccination, immunised animals are protected from disease on challenge with hepatitis B virus (G. Smith, personal communication). Clearly, it will not be long before other cloned virus genes are inserted into vaccinia viruses to make further "generic" vaccines. The fact that vaccinia DNA can tolerate large insertions into nonessential regions of the genome opens up the exciting possibility of making polyvalent live vaccinia recombinants. For viruses infecting the respiratory tract, it is conceivable that recombinant live-attenuated adenoviruses, containing the gene coding for the relevant immunogen, could be constructed in a similar way.

VII. CONCLUSIONS AND PROSPECTS

It might have been more appropriate to call this article gene cloning in virus vaccine research, because so many of the examples seem to involve viruses rather than bacteria or parasites. This is probably because more was known about the structure and replication of viruses before recombinant DNA techniques became available and it was relatively straightforward to apply the techniques to different virus genomes directly. This has not only facilitated the nucleotide sequencing of different virus genomes and genes, from which amino acid sequences have been deduced, but also the study of the expression of virus genes in infected cells as well as the directed expression of virus proteins in *E. coli* and other host cells.

It should be remembered, however, that even though a number of serious diseases are caused by viruses, many of the most devastating infectious diseases involve complex parasites that are difficult or impossible to culture *in vitro,* e.g., malaria, schistosomiasis (bilharzia), filiarisis, and leishmaniasis. It is only recently that the merozoite form of the malarial parasite (*Plasmodium falciparum*) has been cultured in red blood cells. Recombinant DNA techniques are now being used increasingly to investigate parasites and their antigens. Some of the best studied so far are the African trypanosomes (e.g., *Trypanosoma brucei*), which evade the immune system of their host by changing their surface antigens. The molecular basis of this "change of coat", which involves the movement of different surface antigen genes into an "expression site," has been partly unravelled by cloning and sequencing the genes coding for the surface antigens (see Borst and Cross, 1982).

The development of monoclonal antibodies has enabled the major surface antigen of the sporozoite stage of the monkey malaria parasite *Plasmodium knowlesi* to be identified (Kilejian, 1982). These monoclonal antibodies have also been used to select bacteria containing plasmids expressing parts of a cloned sporozoite surface antigen gene. Messenger RNA was extracted from *P. knowlesi*-infected mosquitoes, transcribed into cDNA, and cloned into a plasmid vector, so that a proportion of the plasmids containing surface antigen sequences would be expressed as a fusion protein (Ellis *et al.,* 1983). Nucleotide sequencing of the cDNA now indicates that the sporozoite surface protein has a unique structure; at least one-third of it consists of a 36-base pair (bp) repeat unit. The peptide coded for by this repeat has been synthesised and is being conjugated to various carrier proteins to determine whether antibodies raised by the peptide neutralise the infectivity of *P. knowlesi* sporozoites (Godson *et al.,* 1983).

It would not be surprising to find this sporozoite antigen expressed in different eukaryotic cell vector systems and as a live vaccinia virus recombinant in the coming months. When the gene for the surface antigen of *P. falciparum* sporozoites is cloned, it can then be inserted into whichever system looks the most promising as the basis of a vaccine. Nevertheless, it should be remembered that an effective vaccine against malaria may well have to include antigens from both sporozoite and blood stages of the parasite.

Obviously, not all the approaches to vaccines outlined here will ever become anything more than simply experimental systems. Apart from the expression of the trp LE′ VP1 fusion protein, it is difficult to see *E.coli* being used for the production of virus antigens although it is being used to express bacterial surface components. It is difficult also to envisage the use of peptides for immunisation against foot-and-mouth disease, even if it does prove to be an effective vaccine in protection tests, simply on economic grounds (10^9 doses annually at 1 mg/dose is 1 tonne of peptide). It may be, however, that peptide vaccines will be found useful and economically viable for other virus diseases such as hepatitis A. The production of short peptides as fusion proteins in *E.coli* may be a possible compromise between the peptide and the bacterial expression route. Regions 130–157 and 141–160 of FMDV VP1 expressed this way apparently elicit the formation of neutralising antibodies at a level that should be sufficient to protect against disease (Brown, 1983). Once the characteristics of peptide immunogens are more understood in molecular and configurational terms, it may even be possible to move away from peptides altogether towards totally synthetic vaccines, which mimic the shape of the antigenic determinants.

If subunit vaccines do not effectively stimulate all aspects of the immune response necessary to combat the infection, i.e., both humoral and cell mediated immunity, then "recombinant" live vaccines may well be a realistic alternative. If the expression of HBsAg in yeast and eukaryotic cells is the second generation hepatitis B vaccine then the third generation could be vaccinia virus/ HBsAg recombinants. As hepatitis B is primarily a disease of the underdeveloped world it is certainly attractive to think in terms of a vaccine as cheap to make and as easy to administer and with as few side effects as vaccinia vaccine. The success of the smallpox eradication campaign was not only due to the efficacy of the vaccine but also to its stability and ease of handling under difficult conditions.

Furthermore the availability of other live virus vectors (e.g., adenovirus) may extend the approach to respiratory and enteric virus infections.

One hopes that one or other of these recombinant DNA approaches to the synthesis of various immunogens will form the basis for the vaccines of the future. There is no doubt at all, however, that the information gained about pathogenic microorganisms from the application of recombinant DNA techniques will be useful whatever type of vaccine is being prepared.

ACKNOWLEDGEMENTS

I would like to thank Norman Carey, Spencer Emtage, Gwyn Humphreys and Anita Crafts-Lighty for comments on the manuscript. This chapter is dedicated to my father (the late Dr. Robert Harris), whose enthusiasm kindled my interest in viruses and consequently in recombinant DNA techniques.

REFERENCES

Arnon, R., Shapira, M. and Jacob, C. O. (1983). *J. Immunol. Methods* **61**, 261–273.

Beale, A. J. and Harris, R. J. C. (1979). *Soc. Gen. Microbial. Symp.* **29**, 151–162.

Beggs, J. D. (1981). *In* "Genetic Engineering" (R. Williamson, ed.), Vol. 2, pp. 175–203. Academic Press, London.

Bittle, J. L., Houghton, R. A., Alexander, H., Shinnick, T., Sutcliffe, J. G., Lerner, R. A., Rowlands, D. J. and Brown, F. (1982). *Nature (London)* **298**, 30–33.

Borst, P., and Cross, G. A. M. (1982). *Cell* **29**, 291–303.

Brammar, W. J. (1982). *In* "Genetic Engineering" (R. Williamson, ed.), Vol. 3, pp. 53–81. Academic Press, London.

Brown, F. (1983). *Nature (London)* **304**, 395–396.

Chater, K. F., Hopwood, D., Kiester, T. and Thompson, C. J. (1982). *Curr. Top. Microbiol. Immunol.* **96**, 69–95.

Christman, J., Gerber, M., Price, P. M., Flordellis, C., Edelman, J. and Acs, G. (1982). *Proc. Natl. Acad. Sci. U.S.A.* **79**, 1815–1819.

Clarke, B. E., Carroll, A. R., Rowlands, D. J., Nicholson, B. H., Houghton, R. A., Lerner, R. A. and Brown, F. (1983). *FEBS Letts.* **157**, 261–264.

Davis, A. R., Bos, T., Veda, M., Nayak, D., Dowbenko, D., and Compans, R. W. (1983). *Gene* **21**, 273–284.

Ellis, J., Ozaki, L. S., Gwadz, R. W., Cochrane, A. H., Nussenzweig, V., Nussenzweig, R. and Godson, G. N. (1983). *Nature (London)* **302**, 536–538.

Emini, E. A., Jameson, B. A. and Wimmer, E. (1983). *Nature (London)* **304**, 699–703.

Emtage, J. S., Tacon, W. C. A., Catlin, G. H., Jenkins, B., Porter, A. G. and Carey, N. H. (1980). *Nature (London)* **283**, 171–174.

Evans, D. M. A., Minor, P. D., Schild, G. C. and Almond, J. W. (1983). *Nature (London)* **304**, 409–462.

Fujisawa, Y., Ito, Y., Sasada, R., Ono, Y., Igarashi, K., Marumoto, R., Kikuchi, M. and Sugino, Y. (1983). *Nucleic Acids Res.* **11**, 3581–3591.

Fujiyama, A., Miyanohara, A., Nozaki, C., Yoneyama, T., Ohtomo, N. and Matsubara, K. (1983). *Nucleic Acids Res.* **11**, 4601–4610.

Gerin, J., Alexander, H., Shih, J-W. K., Purcell, R. H., Dapolito, G., Engle, R., Green, N., Sutcliffe, J. G., Shinnick, T. M. and Lerner, R. A. (1983). *Proc. Natl. Acad. Sci. U.S.A.* **80**, 2365–2369.

Gething, M. J. and Sambrook, J. (1981). *Nature (London)* **293**, 620–625.

Gething, M. J. and Sambrook, J. (1982). *Nature (London)* **300**, 598–603.

Godson, G. N., Ellis, J., Schlesinger, D. H., and Nussenzweig, V. (1983). *Nature (London)* **305**, 29–33.

Green, N., Alexander, H., Olson, A., Alexander, S., Shinnick, T. M., Sutcliffe, J. G. and Lerner, R. A. (1982). *Cell* **28**, 477–487.

Harris, T. J. R. (1983). *In* "Genetic Engineering" (R. Williamson, ed.), Vol. 4, pp. 128–175. Academic Press, London.

Hinnen, A. and Meyhack, B. (1982). *Curr. Top. Microbiol. Immunol.* **96**, 101–117.

Hitzeman, R. A., Chen, C. Y., Hagie, F. E., Patzer, E. J., Liu, C. C., Estell, D. A., Miller, J. V., Yaffe, A., Kleid, D. G., Levinson, A. D. and Loppermann, H. (1983). *Nucleic Acids Res.* **11**, 2745–2763.

Hollenberg, C. P. (1982). *Curr. Top. Microbiol. Immunol.* **96**, 119–144.

Kilejian, A. (1982). *Trends Biochem. Sci.* **7**, 5–6.

Kleid, D. G., Yansura, D., Small, D., Dowbenko, D., Moore, D. M., Grubman, M. J., Mckercher, P. D., Morgan, D. O., Robertson, B. H. and Bachrach, H. L. (1981). *Science* **214**, 1125–1129.

Kreft, J., and Hughes, C. (1982). *Curr. Top. Microbiol. Immunol.* **96**, 1–17.

Lamb, R. A. and Choppin, P. W. (1983). *Annu. Rev. Biochem.* **52**, 467–507.

Lerner, R. A. (1982). *Nature (London)* **299**, 592–596.

Lerner, R. A. (1983). *Sci. Am.* **248**, 48–56.

Mackett, M., Smith, G. L. and Moss, B. (1982). *Proc. Natl. Acad. Sci. U.S.A.* **79**, 7415–7419.

Makoff, A. J., Paynter, C., Rowlands, D. J. and Boothroyd, J. C. (1982). *Nucleic Acids Res.* **10**, 8285–8295.

Minor, P. D., Schild, G. C., Bootman, J., Evans, D. M. A., Ferguson, M., Reeve, P., Spitz, M., Stanway, G., Cann, A. J., Hauptmann, R., Clarke, L. D., Mountford, R. C. and Almond, J. W. (1983). *Nature (London)* **301**, 674–679.

Miyanohara, A., Tohe, A., Nozaki, C., Hamada, F., Ohtomo, N. and Matsubara, K. (1983). *Proc. Natl. Acad. Sci. U.S.A.* **80**, 1–5.

Moriarty, A. M., Hoyer, B. H., Shih, J. W., Gerin, J. and Hamer, D. H. (1981). *Proc. Natl. Acad. Sci. U.S.A.* **78**, 2606–2610.

Nomoto, A., Omata, T., Toyoda, H., Kuge, S., Horie, H., Katakoa, Y., Genba, Y., Nakano, Y. and Imura, N. (1982). *Proc. Natl. Acad. Sci. U.S.A.* **79**, 5793–5797.

Norrby, E. (1983). *Arch. Virol.* **76**, 163–177.

Old, R. W. and Primrose, S. B. (1981). "Studies in Microbiology," 2nd ed. Blackwell, Oxford.

Panicali, D. and Paoletti, E. (1982). *Proc. Natl. Acad. Sci. U.S.A.* **79,** 4927–4931.

Panicali, D., Davis, S. W., Weinberg, R. L. and Paoletti, E. (1983). *Proc. Natl. Acad. Sci. U.S.A.* **80,** 5364–5368.

Pfaff, E., Mussgay, M., Bohm, H. O., Schulz, G. E. and Schaller, H. (1982). *EMBO J.* **1,** 869–874.

Racaniello, V. and Baltimore, D. (1981). *Science* **214,** 916–919.

Rigby, P. W. J. (1982). *In* "Genetic Engineering" (R. Williamson, ed.), Vol. 3, pp. 88–141. Academic Press, London.

Rigby, P. W J. (1983). *J. Gen. Virol.* **64,** 255–266.

Sambrook, J. and Grodzicker, T. (1980). *In* "Genetic Engineering: Principles and Methods (J. K. Setlow and A. Hollaender, eds.), Vol. 2, pp. 103–114. Plenum, New York.

Smith, G. L., Mackett, M. and Moss, B. (1983). *Nature (London)* **302,** 490–495.

Stenlund, A., Lamy, D., Moreno-Lopez, J., Ahola, H., Pettersson, U. and Tiollais, P. (1983). *EMBO J.* **2,** 669–673.

Strohmaier, K., Franze, R. and Adam, K-H. (1982). *J. Gen. Virol.* **59,** 295–306.

Sutcliffe, J. G., Shinnick, F. M., Green, N. and Lerner, R. A. (1983). *Science* **219,** 660–666.

Sveda, M. M. and Lai, C. J. (1981). *Proc. Natl. Acad. Sci. U.S.A.* **78,** 5488–5492.

Sveda, M. M., Markoff, L. J. and Lai, C. J. (1982). *Cell* **30,** 649–656.

Tiollais, P., Charnay, P. and Vyas, G. N. (1981). *Science* **213,** 406–411.

Valenzuela, P., Medina, A., Rutter, W. J., Ammerer, G., and Hall, B. D. (1982). *Nature (London)* **298,** 347–350.

Van der Werf, S., Dreano, M., Bruneau, P., Kopecka, H. and Girard, M. (1983). *Gene* **23,** 85–93.

Wang, Y., Stratowa, C., Schaefer-Ridder, M., Doehmer, J. and Hofschneider, P. H. (1983). *Mol. Cell Biol.* **3,** 1032–1039.

Watson, R. J., Weis, J. H., Salstrom, J. S. and Enquist, L. W. (1982). *Science* **218,** 381–384.

Wiley, D. C., Wilson, I. A. and Skehel, J. J. (1981). *Nature (London)* **289,** 373–378.

Williams, J. (1981). *In* "Genetic Engineering" (R. Williamson, ed.), Vol. 1. Academic Press, London.

Wunner, W. H., Dietzschold, B., Curtis, P. J. and Wiktor, T. J. (1983). *J. Gen. Virol.* **64,** 1649–1656.

Yelverton, E., Norton, S., Obijeski, J. F. and Goeddel, D. V. (1983). *Science* **219,** 614–619.

Zoller, M. and Smith, M. (1982). *Nucleic Acids Res.* **10,** 6487–6500.

Zuckerman, A. J. (1982). *Br. Med. J.* **284,** 686–688.

4

Synthetic Vaccines

RUTH ARNON

Department of Chemical Immunology,
The Weizmann Institute of Science,
Rehovot, Israel

I. INTRODUCTION

Ever since the times of Jenner and Pasteur, vaccination has been accepted as a part of our way of life and constitutes one of the most successful achievements in the field of immunology. Indeed, existing vaccines are highly rewarding in providing immunity against many infectious diseases, and even the eradication of some. However, there are several drawbacks to the vaccination procedures that are presently used, especially those concerning viral vaccines.

IMMUNE INTERVENTION
Copyright © 1984 by Academic Press, London
All rights of reproduction in any form reserved
ISBN 0-12-593301-0

It is of some interest that real advances in the development of antiviral vaccines have always been the result of a major breakthrough. The first breakthrough occurred at the end of the seventeenth century when Jenner introduced vaccination with cowpox virus to protect against smallpox. This was the first attempt at active immunization. Almost a century passed before the second breakthrough, which was the first to be based on an immunological principle; this breakthrough was Pasteur's use of attenuation of a virus by passage in a new host, which led to the rabies vaccine. Following this development, the major problem then became how to grow the viruses. The next breakthrough was in the use of the embryonated egg for this purpose, which led to the development of several other vaccines, such as yellow fever and influenza. The cell culture technique was the next breakthrough, and it resulted in the production of additional vaccines, such as polio and measles.

Because of existing vaccines, various kinds of infectious or communicable diseases have been diminished in their incidence and importance. However, concomitantly new diseases, caused by other viruses or by different strains of the same viruses, are replacing them, and this is the reason why new vaccines are required continuously. Further breakthroughs in this field are required now, probably through the use of molecular biology or, possibly, a synthetic approach such as the one discussed in this chapter.

Before attempting to synthesize a vaccine, we should be clear about the exact criteria for its evaluation. Vaccination, in general, involves the use of an immunizing agent, which is expected to elicit protection, namely, the formation of neutralizing antibodies or cytotoxic cells against a biologically active material, such as a bacterium, virus, or toxin. The immunizing agent comprises usually the intact organism, but as shown for simpler biologically active molecules, such as enzymes, only a small fraction of the elicited antibodies possess the entire neutralizing capacity. The questions we face are therefore threefold: (1) Is it possible to identify the antigenic region(s) in a biologically active material that participate in the neutralizing process? (2) Is it possible to induce an immune response with exclusive specificity for such determinants? (3) Is it possible to synthesize a molecule analogous to such a region that will, in turn, lead to efficient protective immunity? Positive answers to these three questions provided the essential steps for the production of synthetic vaccines, as will be described in the following sections.

II. IDENTIFICATION OF ANTIGENIC DETERMINANTS

The important components in the induction of immunity, especially viral immunity, are proteins and glycoproteins; what do we know about their immunological properties? This subject was discussed in detail in the review by Arnon and Geiger (1977). Essentially, in the course of an immune response, these antigens exhibit two distinct reactivities, which may not necessarily coincide. The first is *immunogenicity,* that is, the capacity of the antigenic material to elicit an immune response manifested either by antibody production or by cell-medicated immunity. The second characteristic, *antigenic specificity,* refers to the antigen's capacity to react in a specific manner with antibodies or with immune lymphocytes, regardless of how these have been produced. The regions in the antigen molecule that come into direct contact with the active site of the antibodies or with the cell receptors are defined as *antigenic determinants.*

Macromolecules may carry a large number and variety of possible antigenic determinants that dictate their antigenic specificity. However, only a limited number of the potential antigenic sites are important for the immunogenicity, i.e., are immunodominant. In viral antigens, an even smaller number of determinants are involved in inducing neutralizing immunity. The parameters found to be most important for the immunological properties are the molecular size of the immunogen, the spatial conformation, and the accessibility of the antigenic determinants. The *molecular size* is important primarily for immunogenicity, presumably because the larger the molecule the greater the number of potential determinants, particularly potential "carrier" determinants required for T helper cell involvement. Small molecules are often nonimmunogenic, but they can be made immunogenic by coupling to carriers. Consequently, coupling is a common procedure employed in the preparation of synthetic vaccines. The accessibility of the determinant is a crucial factor because the interaction of any individual antigenic determinant with either the antibodies or specific receptors of the immunocompetent cells necessitates its exposure on the antigenic molecule. As a result, in many native proteins, antigenic determinants consist of segments that are at the "corners" of the folded polypeptide chain and are fully or partly exposed on the surface of the protein molecule.

The *spatial conformation* of proteins plays a decisive role in determining the antigenic specificity. As discussed in detail by Crumpton (1974) and Arnon (1974), there is cumulative evidence that a drastic change in antigenic properties occurs upon denaturation of native proteins or by unfolding their polypeptide chains. But, in many instances, more subtle conformational alterations are also accompanied by a change in the antigenic reactivity; the best example of such systems concerns the change in antigenicity associated with removal of the haem group from spermwhale myoglobin (Crumpton and Wilkinson, 1966). Antibodies specific for the haem-free apomyoglobin can react with the intact metmyoglobin, but induce in it a conformational change that causes the release of the haem group during the antigen–antibody interaction. This observation, and many others, have led to the conclusion that most of the antigenic determinants of proteins are *conformational determinants,* namely, they result from the three-dimensional steric configuration and may include residues that are distal in the unfolded peptide chain but occupy juxtapositions in the native molecule. Antibodies specific towards such determinants will not necessarily react with isolated peptides derived from the molecule, whereas antibodies directed against *sequential determinants* will usually recognize stretches of amino acid sequences in the protein and react with short peptide fragments of it (Sela *et al.*, 1967).

Identification of antigenic determinants is usually accomplished by fragmentation of the native protein either by chemical cleavage adjacent to specific residues or by controlled proteolysis. The resultant fragments are then screened for immunologically active components that can bind to the antibodies and interfere with their interaction with the intact antigen. In that manner, defined determinants have been localized in several protein molecules, as demonstrated in the following examples:

1. *Tobacco mosaic virus protein (TMVP).* This protein is the only constitutent of the protein coat of tobacco mosaic virus; it

consists of one polypeptide chain of 158 amino acid residues, the sequence of which is known (Tsugita *et al.,* 1960). Immunochemical studies with this protein demonstrated that an icosapeptide, comprising the residues 93–112 of the protein, possesses the total inhibitory activity of a tryptic digest and thus encompasses the single antigenic determinant of the protein. Furthermore, most of the activity resides in its three terminal residues Ala-Thr-Arg (Benjamini *et al.,* 1969).

2. *Sperm whale myoglobin* is a protein for which the full antigenic mapping has been accomplished using several approaches and methodologies. The data, in this case as well, indicate that a relatively large proportion of the antimyoglobin antibody population is directed towards a comparatively small portion of the total surface of the antigen. Five independent determinants have been identified, and as shown in Fig. 1, all of them are localized at the corners of the molecule that separate the helical regions. All these defined determinants are small, consisting of only five to seven amino acid residues, but they are all exposed on the surface of the molecule (Attasi, 1975).

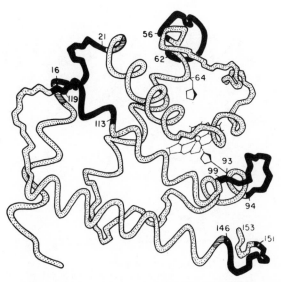

Fig. 1.   A schematic diagram showing the mode of folding of myoglobin with the antigenic determinants in black. (From Attasi, 1975.)

3. *Hen egg-white lysozyme* is the last example to be mentioned here. Two independent antigenic regions have been identified in this protein; both are conformation dependent and contain disulfide bonds that stabilize the structure and are crucial for the antigenic specificity. One of these defined determinants contains the C-and N-terminal segments linked by a disulfide bond, whereas the second is a larger region, comprising residues 57–104 and containing two disulfide bonds. This region can be further split to yield a smaller immunologically active peptide with the amino acid sequence 60–83, containing a single disulfide bond between cysteines 64 and 80, which is described as the "loop" (Arnon and Sela, 1969). From the three-dimensional structure of lysozyme (Fig. 2), it becomes clear that this region is exposed on the surface of the molecule. Studies with antibodies specific for the loop (Maron *et al.*, 1971;

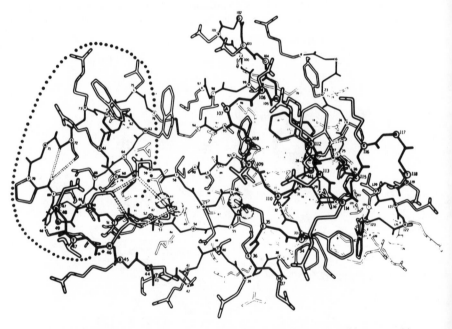

Fig. 2.   A schematic diagram of the three-dimensional structure of hen egg-white lysozyme according to the "Atlas of Protein Sequence and Structure" (M. O. Dayhoff, ed.) and the location of the "loop" antigenic determinant, identified by the dotted line. (From Arnon, 1974.)

Pecht *et al.*, 1971) demonstrated that it is a conformation-dependent determinant.

III. SYNTHETIC ANTIGENS WITH PROTEIN SPECIFICITY

Once an antigenic determinant in a protein has been identified, the present methodology in peptide and polymer synthesis enables its chemical synthesis. As a consequence, synthetic peptides or their conjugates with macromolecular carriers can be investigated and characterized for their immunological properties. This approach has been employed in the case of several protein antigens, as exemplified in the following.

The first example is *collagen,* the protein constituent of connective tissue and probably the most abundant protein in animals. The collagen of vertebrates is composed of three polypeptide chains: two identical α_1 chains and one α_2 chain, which are supercoiled in the form of a characteristic triple helix. Collagen as such is a weak immunogen, and immunization with the native protein leads mainly to antibodies directed towards the N- and C-terminal nonhelical regions of both types of chains, which show considerable interspecies differences. The helical region of collagen has been conserved during evolution to a greater extent than other parts, yet some interspecies differences have been observed in this region as well, and they are expressed in some conformation-dependent antigenic determinants. This assumption was indirectly confirmed by the synthetic approach: A synthetic periodic polypeptide (Pro-Gyl-Pro)$_n$, which was shown to have a collagen-like triple-helical structure (Traub and Yonath, 1966), was found to be immunogenic in guinea pigs (Borek *et al.,* 1969). Immunization with this co-polymer elicited antibodies that, in addition to their reaction with the homologous polymer, reacted also with native collagens (Fig. 3) of several species (Fuchs *et al.,* 1974), leading to a quasi-autoimmune phenomena. This cross-reaction is by virtue of the triple-helical conformation, which is common to the synthetic material and the various collagens.

In the case of hen egg-white lysozyme, the loop determinant (residues 60–83) described earlier has been chemically synthesized, using the solid phase peptide synthesis method of Merrifield

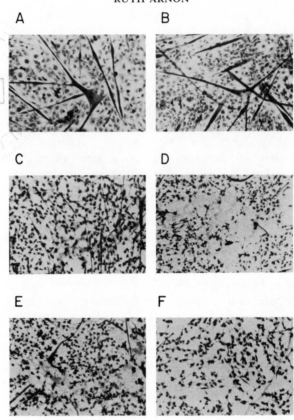

Fig. 3. Effect of antisera on rat muscle cells. (A) Normal muscle cells; (B) cells incubated with complement alone; (C and D) cells exposed to anti-acid-soluble rat tail collagen at 1000-fold and 100-fold dilutions; (E and F) cells exposed to anti-(pro-gly-pro)$_n$ antibodies (4 μg/ml). (From Fuchs *et al.*, 1974.)

(1965) and was attached to a synthetic carrier. The resultant completely synthetic conjugate elicited antibodies that were reactive with native lysozyme and could still recognize the conformation-dependent determinant in the intact molecule (Arnon *et al.*, 1971). Furthermore, an obvious advantage of the synthetic approach is that, once an active derivative is identified, many analogs can be synthesized and used for detailed analysis of the antigenic specificity and the elucidation of the parameters responsible for such activity. Indeed, investigation of several analogs of the lysozyme loop peptide, in which one or two residues were replaced by alanine, revealed that a major role is played by specific amino acid residues, in particular proline, in the antigenic reactivity of this determinant (Teicher *et al.*, 1973).

The last example is a protein of great interest, namely, the carcinoembryonic antigen (CEA) of the colon. This glycoprotein of about 200,000 daltons is characteristic of many types of cancer tissues, and antibodies against it are used in a radioimmunoassay for detection of cancer. The synthetic approach has been employed in this case as well: a peptide corresponding to the 11 amino acid residues of the NH_2-terminal portion of the sequence of CEA, denoted CEA (1–11), has been synthesized and chemically attached both to a synthetic carrier and to bovine serum albumin. Both macromolecular conjugates evoked antipeptide antibodies in rabbits. Investigation of the specificity of this immunological system has revealed that the peptide reacted not only with its homologous antibodies but also with anti-CEA sera. Likewise, the antiserum against the peptide reacted with intact CEA (Arnon *et al.*, 1976).

These examples clearly demonstrate that, once an immunologically reactive region in a protein is identified, it can be synthesized and used for the induction of antibodies that react with the intact protein in its native form. The spatial conformation plays an important role in this activity.

IV. SYNTHETIC PEPTIDES AS A BASIS FOR FUTURE VACCINES

As evident from the previous section, although most antigenic determinants of proteins are thought to be conformational rather than sequential, relatively short peptide segments that are exposed on the surface or at ''corners'' of the spatial structure, constitute major antigenic determinants. Furthermore, synthetic antigens that contain such immunoreactive region(s) can give rise to an immune response towards the intact molecule. There is no reason why this should be limited to soluble proteins. It should be feasible to use a similar approach for components of viruses or bacteria, with the purpose of inducing antibodies reactive with the intact organism and hopefully leading to its neutralization. As will be discussed in Section IV, A–F, several examples in the recent literature prove that this goal is indeed within reach.

A. Tobacco Mosaic Virus

The first report of a peptide fragment that induced an antiviral response was by Anderer (1963a), who described his work on tobacco mosaic virus (TMV). This virus is a rod-like particle of molecular weight 40×10^6 and is composed of a 5% RNA core surrounded by a coat of 2200 identical protein subunits that form 95% of the virus and are packed in a characteristic ordered pattern (Fig. 4). The interaction of TMV with antiserum raised against the intact virus results in neutralization of the virus infectivity. Anderer observed that peptides isolated from enzymatic digests of TMV protein had the capacity to partially inhibit the quantitative precipitation of the TMV by its rabbit antibodies. In this interaction, the

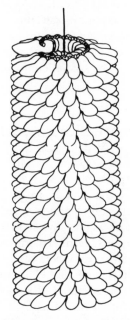

Fig. 4.   Diagram of the tobacco mosaic virus. (From Caspar, 1963).

icosapeptide, which is immunologically active in the TMV protein system, was not inhibitory. The only immunologically active region of the TMV protein in the interaction of the whole virus with the antibodies was the C-terminal hexapeptide. This phenomenon is probably due to the exclusive exposure of this peptide on the surface of the virus, as a result of the packing of the protein subunits around the RNA core.

Based on these findings, Anderer (1963b) isolated the C-terminal hexapeptide Thr-Ser-Gly-Pro-Ala-Thr from TMV protein enzymatic digest, attached it to bovine serum albumin, and used the resultant conjugate for the immunization of rabbits. The antiserum contained antibodies that precipitated with the homologous antigen, as well as (although to a much lesser extent) with the intact tobacco mosaic virus. The most important observation of that study, as emphasized by Anderer, was that the antiserum raised towards the artificial conjugate, when mixed in large excess with tobacco mosaic virus, partially inhibited the appearance of lesions when it was applied to tobacco plants, namely the infectivity of the virus.

Although the hexapeptide used in this study was obtained from an enzyme digest of the *native* protein, it can still be considered within the realm of synthetic materials, because such short peptides can now be easily prepared by chemical synthesis. The drawback of this system, however, is the limited antiviral immune response of the antipeptide antibodies (as compared to anti-TMV antibodies) in neutralizing the infectivity of the virus.

B. MS-2 Coliphage—A Model Viral System

In a more recent study, using the model system of the coliphage MS-2, an immunologically active synthetic peptide was described, which induced antibodies capable of *efficiently* neutralizing the native bacteriophage. This virus is infective in *E. coli* bacteria and causes their complete lysis, a phenomenon that is manifested in the formation of virus plaques on monolayers of bacteria (Fig. 5A). The MS-2 phage is an RNA-containing virus with icosahedral symmetry (Fig. 6). The viral capsid contains 180 identical coat-protein subunits, with a molecular weight of 13,000, each coat-protein subunit consisting of a single polypeptide chain with known sequence (Liu *et al.*, 1967; Weber and Koenigsberg, 1975). Anti-

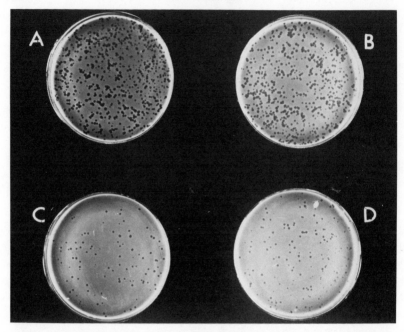

Fig. 5.   MS-2 coliphage and its neutralization by specific antisera. The plaques of the MS-2 phage are visible as small clear zones in the opaque layer of growing *E. coli* bacteria. (A) MS-2 phage in buffer; (B) after incubation with normal rabbit serum; (C) after incubation with anti-MS-2 serum; (D) after incubation with antiserum against the synthetic P_2-A--L.

sera prepared against the total phage or even against the monomeric units of the coat proteins are efficient in neutralizing the intact phage and thus in decreasing the number of its plaques (Fig. 5C). Efforts were, therefore, made to locate and identify the regions(s) in the molecule that participate in the immunological activity and in the neutralizing process, in order to explore the possibility of using synthetic materials that would provoke neutralizing antibodies. For that purpose, the coat protein was cleaved with cyanogen bromide, a simple chemical agent known to split protein chains only near the amino acid methionine, and the resulting fragments were screened for their capacity to inhibit the neutralization of the phage by antiphage antibodies. In accordance with the amino acid sequence of the coat protein, three fragments were obtained: one

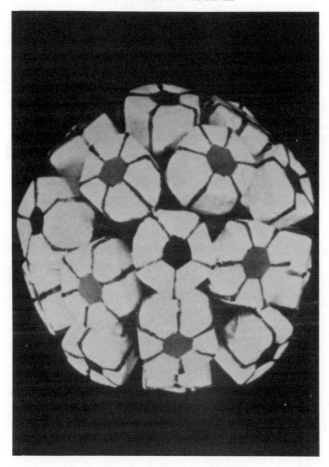

Fig. 6.   A model of MS-2 coliphage. (From Vasquez *et al.*, 1966.)

fragment of about 10,000 daltons and two fragments each of about 2000 daltons.

The mixture of the two small fragments, P_2 and P_3, was found capable of inhibiting the neutralization of the phage by antiserum to the whole MS-2, almost to the same degree as the intact native protein, indicating that at least one of them is involved in the phage neutralization. In order to evaluate the synthetic approach, the two peptides were synthesized. The synthetic P_3, corresponding to the carboxy-terminal 21 amino acid residues in the sequence of the coat protein, had no activity whatsoever. On the other hand, the synthetic P_2 peptide was very efficient in inhibiting the inactivation of phage by the antiserum against the phage. Furthermore, a synthetic antigen, prepared by attachment of P_2 covalently to poly-DL-alanyl poly-L-lysine and denoted P_2-A—L, induced antibodies in rabbits that were capable of neutralizing MS-2 activity almost as efficiently as the antibodies against the intact coat protein (Fig. 5D). These results provided the first reported evidence that a synthetic peptide could be utilized for eliciting antiviral responses (Langbeheim *et al.*, 1976).

C. Effect of Adjuvant

An important consideration in all vaccines is the adjuvant they contain in order to augment the immunogenicity of the primary agent. This point is even more crucial when synthetic vaccines are considered, since most of these substances are water soluble and tend to be less immunogenic than particulate materials. For experimental immunization in laboratory animals, the most commonly used adjuvant is Freund's complete adjuvant (FCA), which contains killed mycobacteria dispersed in water-in-oil emulsion (Freund, 1947). It usually evokes high-level and long-lasting immunity. This adjuvant, however, is too problematic and is not adequate for use in humans, because it induces local reactions, probably due to the very slow metabolic removal, if any, of the mineral oil and to the inflammation caused by the mycobacteria. Efforts are being made to replace the mineral oil with mixtures of readily metabolizable components or to eliminate it completely and replace the mycobacteria by less damaging materials.

The minimal adjuvant active structure that can substitute for mycobacteria in Freund's complete adjuvant is synthetic N-acetylmuramyl-L-alanyl-D-isoglutamine (or MDP for muramyl dipeptide) (Ellouz *et al.*, 1974; Kotani *et al.*, 1975). Contrary to other mycobacterial fractions, MDP is an active adjuvant when administered in aqueous medium parenterally or even orally. For this reason, MDP was used to investigate the augmentation of the antigenicity of P_2-A—L. The results showed that when mixed with the P_2-A—L, the MDP had only limited adjuvant effect. However, when it was covalently attached, the resulting MDP-P_2-A—L conjugate elicited in rabbits, when administered in phosphate buffered saline, almost as good an anti-MS-2 response as did the immunization of P_2-A—L in complete Freund's adjuvant (Arnon *et al.*, 1980).

This finding as such is of great importance, because it indicates that it is possible to design a completely synthetic vaccine, containing synthetic carrier, synthetic determinant, and synthetic adjuvant. Such a vaccine has built-in adjuvanticity and hence is effective in providing immunity even when administered in physiological saline.

D. Diphtheria Toxin

These successful results prompted the search for other systems in which the synthetic approach could be applied. One example is diphtheria toxin, which is excreted by the diphtheria bacillus and is the component responsible for its toxic effect. Its activity can be demonstrated experimentally by a dermonecrotic effect in the skin of animals at the site of injection. The toxin consists of a single polypeptide chain of 62,000 daltons with two disulfide bridges. Vaccination against diphtheria is achieved by immunization with the detoxified toxin, or toxoid, antibodies against which also react with the native toxin and neutralize its toxicity. Audibert *et al.* (1982) have shown that active antitoxic immunization against diphtheria could also be achieved by a synthetic peptide attached to a protein carrier. This peptide, a tetradecapeptide (denoted STDP) consists of the residues 188–201 in the amino acid sequence of diphtheria toxin and represents a fragment of the disulfide loop that comprises the two functional segments of the natural diphtheria toxin molecule. Conjugates of this peptide, or the hexapeptide 186–201, linked covalently to either proteins or a synthetic carrier, elicited antibodies in guinea pigs that not only bound specifically with the toxin, but also neutralized its dermonecrotic activity and lethal effect.

Furthermore, in a more recent study (Audibert *et al.*, 1982), it was shown that as in the case of the MS-2 bacteriophage, a completely synthetic conjugate comprising the hexapeptide of the toxin sequence and MDP, covalently attached to the synthetic carrier multichain poly DL-alanine, induced a most effective immune response in mice. This is the first report on a completely synthetic immunogen with built-in adjuvanticity, which induces protective antitoxic immunity when administered in a physiological medium.

E. LHRH—A Synthetic Vaccine for Immunological Castration

The release of luteinizing hormone (LH) and of follicle stimulating hormone (FSH) have been shown to be under the control of a decapeptide called LH releasing hormone (LHRH). Immunization against this hormone could offer an experimental tool and also a veterinary vaccine for increasing meat production by immunological castration. This hormone, mainly in its synthetic form, has been used for immunization, and indeed it led to neutralization of the LHRH activity in several animal species. Being a weak immunogen, this process required repeated immunizations or the use of highly immunogenic protein carrier and a strong adjuvant such as complete Freund's adjuvant.

Recently, Carelli *et al.* (1982) have shown that a completely synthetic vaccine can be employed in this system as well. Thus, when the synthetic decapeptide LHRH was directly conjugated to a lysine derivative of MDP, the resultant conjugate yielded high titers of anti LHRH antibodies in mice and led to atrophy of spermatozoides as well. These results are encouraging for practical purposes, but they also serve as another step in the general direction of synthetic vaccines.

F. *Streptococcus pyogenes* M Protein

Streptococcus pyogenes is an organism responsible for widely distributed infections that are also the cause of many complications such as rheumatic fever. The M protein is one of its surface components, and it exhibits sequence variation in different types of streptococci. One of the functions of the M protein is to enable the organism to resist ingestion and killing by phagocytic cells in the blood of the nonimmune host. In the immune host, type-specific antibodies against the M protein neutralize the antiphagocytic effect and allow rapid elimination of any invading streptococci having the same serotype as the M protein. Studies on the primary structure of one of the M proteins (type 24) have indicated that the molecule is composed of repeating covalent structures, each of which contains protective antigenic determinants (Beachy *et al.*, 1978). These results suggested that only a small portion of the M protein molecule may be required to produce primary protective immunity. This notion was recently confirmed by the synthetic approach: a 35-amino acid residue peptide corresponding to the sequence of a fragment of the M protein has been synthesized. Rabbits immunized with this peptide emulsified in complete Fruend's adjuvant mounted both cellular and humoral immune responses to the intact M protein. Moreover, passive immunization of mice with sera of these rabbits provided protection against a challenge infection with type 24 streptococci (Beachy *et al.*, 1981). These results could lead to the development of M protein vaccines to protect against streptococcal infections, which carry the risk of acute rheumatic fever and rheumatic heart disease.

V. SYNTHETIC ANTIVIRAL VACCINES

The key question is whether synthetic peptides could serve as a basis for really practical viral vaccines, particularly in cases in which the existing vaccines are not good or safe enough or where it is difficult to grow the virus in culture for vaccine preparation. The results obtained recently for three such viral systems, namely, hepatitis B, influenza, and foot-and-mouth disease are rather encouraging.

A. Hepatitis B

Hepatitis B virus cannot readily be grown in culture, and, therefore, the only material available for vaccine preparation is the surface antigen (HBsAg) obtained from the blood of chronic human carriers. As a result, the existing vaccine against hepatitis B is not readily available and is very expensive. Hence, this is probably one of the most important systems for which the synthetic approach might provide a satisfactory answer if successful results are obtained.

Three research groups have employed this strategy and each has focused on different sites on the HBsAg molecule as being crucial for the immune response:

Lerner and his colleagues synthesized thirteen peptides corresponding to amino acid sequences predicted from the nucleotide sequence of the HBsAg DNA, and covering most of its 220 residues (Lerner et al., 1981). The free or carrier (KLH)-linked synthetic peptides were injected into rabbits and 7 of the 13 elicited an antipeptide response. Antisera against four of the six soluble peptides that are longer than 10 amino acids were reactive with the native antigen and specifically precipitated the 23,000 and 28,000 dalton forms from Dane particles of the virus. The most effective peptide corresponded to the sequence 95–109. However, the authors do not indicate whether the antibodies it elicited can neutralize the virus or whether the conjugate provides protection against infection.

Melnick and his colleagues (Dreesman et al., 1982) have used another approach. Rather than synthesizing a whole series of peptides, they chose one region that, according to their prediction (based upon computer analyzed secondary structure and hydrophobicity), should be exposed on the intact particle and consequently would represent a potentially exposed antigenic determinant. This region, which contains an internal disulfide "loop," consists of the amino acid sequence 117–137. Two cyclic peptides of this region containing disulfide bonds were synthesized, both of them unrelated to any of Lerner's peptides. These peptides, without linkage to a carrier and upon the use of various adjuvants, elicited an antibody response in mice after a single injection. However, in this case as well, the immune response was established by a radioimmunoassay, with no indication as to the neutralizing capacity of the provoked antibodies.

The third and most recent report concerning the hepatitis B virus is that of Vyas and his colleagues (Bhatnagar et al., 1982). These authors synthesized seven peptide analogs of HBsAg, linked them to KLH, and immunized rabbits with the conjugates. They checked the antigenicity of each peptide by serologic neutralization of human antibodies specific for the a determinant of HBsAg. Three of the analogs obtained from the same region of the molecule (sequences 139–147, 139–158, and 140–158) reacted with preformed antibody and were able to induce anti-HBsAg. These results indicated to the authors that the nonapeptide sequence 139–147 represents the total or an essential part of the a determinant of HBsAg, which is common to all stereotypes of the virus. It is still not indicated whether the antibodies formed are neutralizing for the virus or whether immunization with the conjugates provides protection against infection.

It is, therefore, clear that, in view of the promising results, this system requires further research and development.

B. Foot-and-Mouth Disease

In the case of foot-and-mouth disease, the situation is different. Although some strains are still difficult to grow in sufficiently high titer, an existing vaccine is available that is efficient and also inexpensive. The main advantage of a synthetic vaccine in such competition is its safety—a few outbreaks of foot-and-mouth disease have been associated with failures of the virus inactivation process. A synthetic vaccine is, of course, completely safe from this point of view and can overcome such problems. Hence, an effort in this direction has been made, using both cloning of the virus genome and chemical synthesis of fragments of its proteins. Of tremendous help in these efforts was the extensive knowledge of this virus, including its structure, antigenic variants and mechanism of replication (Brown, 1981). The virus particles consist of one molecule of infectious single stranded RNA, and 60 copies of each of 4 structural polypeptides VP1–VP4 (Fig. 7). VP1 was shown to be of antigenic importance, although in the isolated form it is a weak immunogen. Nevertheless, chemically synthesized fragments of this protein have recently been prepared, and their conjugates to KLH were tested as immunogens for inducing a reponse against the intact virus (Bittle et al., 1982).

The sequence of the peptides to be synthesized was predicted from the viral nucleotide sequence, and peptides corresponding to three different regions in the VP1 were prepared. Peptides of two regions produced high levels of serotype-specific virus neutralizing antibodies in cattle, guinea pigs, and rabbits. All these antisera reacted in the immunoprecipitation technique with the virus native

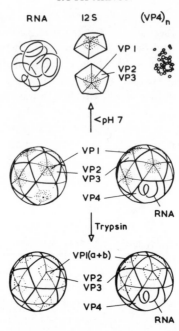

Fig. 7.   Model of foot-and-mouth disease virus. (From Brown, 1981.)

structural proteins and their precursor molecules, which indicates that their specificity resembles that of antiviral sera. Moreover, a single inoculation of the synthetic peptide 141–160 elicited sufficient neutralizing antibody to protect guinea pigs against subsequent challenge with foot-and-mouth disease virus, with an efficiency of 1 to 10% of that of the inactivated virus particle if based on an equal weight basis. Interestingly, the neutralizing antibody titer elicited by the single peptide is several orders of magnitudes greater than the best results obtained with the whole VP1 protein, which was shown to elicit antibodies specific mainly toward the denatured form of the protein. It is thus possible that an entire protein isolated from a virus does not fold properly when deprived of the scaffolding provided by the other structural proteins, whereas a single, relatively short peptide may have better prospects as an appropriate immunogen. These results are, therefore, an important thrust to the notion of totally synthetic vaccines.

C. Influenza Virus

Influenza virus is the third animal virus system with which the synthetic approach for vaccination has been attempted. In this case, the necessity for a novel approach stems from two reasons: (1) The safety consideration—the incidence of Guillain–Barré syndrome appearing in association with the administration of the swine flu vaccine—emphasized the risks involved in the mass use of live influenza vaccines. (2) The rapid changes in the strains and the existence of numerous types and subtypes of the virus, which are serologically distinct. Very often, it can be predicted that any vaccine already developed will not be protective against next year's strain. If a synthetic "multivalent" vaccine that elicits cross-strain protection could be prepared, it would certainly remove an important stumbling block in the development of an optimal, safe and efficient anti-influenza vaccine. Recent reports from our laboratory (Müller *et al.*, 1982; Arnon *et al.*, 1982) show promising results.

A peptide corresponding to the region 91–108 in the amino acid sequence of the hemagglutinin of H3N2-type influenza has been synthesized. This region, which is common to at least nine strains of influenza, is a part of a fragment that had been shown by Jackson *et al.* (1979) to be immunologically active. According to our prediction, it should have comprised a folded "corner" in the three-dimensional conformation and hence an exposed area in the molecular structure, with a favorable chance for having an immunological imprint. Indeed, a conjugate of this peptide with tetanus toxoid elicited antibodies in both rabbits and mice that reacted immunochemically with the peptide as well as with the intact influenza virus of several strains of the subtype A. Moreover, these antibodies were capable of inhibiting the capacity of the hemagglutinin of the relevant strains to agglutinate chicken red blood cells and to interfere with the *in vitro* growth of the virus in tissue culture. Most importantly, mice immunized with the peptide–toxoid conjugate were partially protected against further challenge infection with several strains of the influenza subtype A virus.

As indicated, one of the crucial factors concerning the influenza vaccine is the tremendous genetic variation among the viral strains and its reflection in their serologic differences. The sequences of the hemagglutinins from several strains have been completely determined, and particular amino acid changes correlated with the antigenic differences, whereas other regions were shown to be "constant." We have deliberately chosen part of a preserved sequence, and indeed it elicited a cross-strain protective effect. With the recent elucidation of the three-dimensional structure of the molecule (Wiley *et al.*, 1981), it was of interest to note that this segment of the molecule is exposed on the surface of the hemagglutinin spike and that it is adjacent to a designated antigenic determinant of the molecule that is reactive with neutralizing antibodies.

VI. CONCLUDING REMARKS

It is obvious that if the idea of synthetic vaccine production materializes, it will have tremendous advantages. Synthesis of materials that incorporate peptides consisting of the relevant antigenic determinants of several different viruses and/or bacteria in their structure may lead to multivalent vaccines that will be effective simultaneously towards all these pathogens. It will be possible to build adjuvanticity into the vaccines and thus overcome a serious problem in the production of existing vaccines. It may be possible to take advantage of our knowledge about the genetic control of the immune response and its linkage to the major histocompatibility complex for the design of synthetic vaccines taylored to individuals according to their HLA type. In a paper at the 1972 "Oholo" Conference on "Immunity to Viral and Rickettial Diseases", I stated: "By adequate molecular engineering, all the possible variations of vaccines may be designed, enabling us to have on the shelf a series of different multivalent synthetic vaccines to be used according to a preprogrammed key. This certainly sounds today like a dream. However, with the increasing pace of accumulation of knowledge . . . this dream may become a reality" (Arnon, 1972).

Now, 10 years later, the key question is, of course, whether synthetic peptides can form the basis for *practical* vaccines. The results obtained so far, as summarized above, show great promise. Problems still remain to be solved, however, some generally applicable to all potential vaccines and others more specific to particular vaccines. The feasibility of production of relevant peptides of each and every virus, as well as the economics of synthetic vaccines are also not easy to predict. Whether chemical synthesis is the optimum procedure or whether genetic engineering should be employed for the synthesis is another important consideration. Certainly more knowledge is required on the nature and structure of the proteins involved in the process of neutralization of viruses or on their corresponding viral nucleotide sequences. Nonetheless, the progress made in this direction during the last few years in many laboratories around the world undoubtedly brings the dream of synthetic vaccines nearer reality.

REFERENCES

Anderer, F. A. (1963a). *Naturforsch. Teil B* **18**, 1010–1014.

Anderer, F. A. (1963b). *Biochim. Biophys. Acta* **71**, 246–248.

Arnon, R. (1972). *In* Immunity in Viral and Rickettsial Diseases'' (A. Kohn and M. A. Klinberg, eds.), pp. 209–222. Plennum, New York.

Arnon, R. (1974). *In* "Peptides Polypeptides and Proteins'' (E. R. Blout, F. A. Bovey, M. Goodman and N. Lotan, eds.), pp. 538–553. Wiley, New York.

Arnon, R. and Geiger, B. (1977). *In* "Immunochemistry'' (L. E. Glynn, ed.), pp. 307–363. Wiley, New York.

Arnon, R. and Sela, M. (1969). *Proc. Natl. Acad. Sci. U.S.A.* **62**, 163–170.

Arnon, R., Maron, E., Sela, M. and Anfinsen, C. B. (1971). *Proc. Natl. Acad. Sci. U.S.A.* **68**, 1450–1455.

Arnon, R., Bustin, M., Calef, E., Chaitchik, S., Haimovich, J., Novik, N. and Sela, M. (1976). *Proc. Natl. Acad. Sci. U.S.A.* **73**, 2123–2127.

Arnon, R., Sela, M., Parant, M. and Chedid, L. (1980). *Proc. Natl. Acad. Sci. U.S.A.* **77**, 6769–6772.

Arnon, R., Jibson, M., Müller, G. and Shapira, M. (1982). "International Conference on Immunopharmacology.'' Pergamon, Oxford (in press).

Attasi, M. Z. (1975). *Immunochemistry* **12**, 423–438.

Audibert, F., Jolivet, M., Chedid, L., Alouf, J. E., Boquet, P., Rivaille, P. and Siffert, O. (1981). *Nature (London)* **289**, 593–594.

Audibert, F., Jolivet, M. Chedid, L., Arnon, R. and Sela, M. (1982). *Proc. Natl. Acad. Sci. U.S.A.* **79**, 5042–5046.

Beachy, E. H., Seyer, J. M. and Kang, A. H. (1978). *Proc. Natl. Acad. Sci. U.S.A.* **75**, 3163–3167.

Beachy, E. H., Seyer, J. M., Dale, J. B., Simpson, W. A. and Kang, A. H. (1981). *Nature (London)* **292**, 457–459.

Benjamini, E., Shimizu, M., Young, J. D. and Lenny, C. Y. (1969). *Biochemistry* **8**, 2242–2246.

Bhatnagar, P. K., Papas, E., Blum, H. E., Milich, D. R., Nitecki, D., Karels, M. J. and Vyas, G. N. (1982). *Proc. Natl. Acad. Sci. U.S.A.* **79**, 4400–4404.

Bittle, J. L., Houghten, R. H., Alexander, H., Shinnick, T. H., Sutcliffe, J. G., Lerner, R. A., Rowlands, D. J. and Brown, F. (1982). *Nature (London)* **298**, 30–33.

Borek, F., Kurtz, J. and Sela, M. (1969). *Biochim. Biophys. Acta.* **188**, 314–323.

Brown, F. (1981). *TIBS,* pp. 325–327.

Carelli, C., Audibert, F., Gaillard, J. and Chedid, L. (1982). *Int. J. Immunopharmacol.* **4**, 290.

Caspar, D. L. D. (1963). *Adv. Prot. Chem.* **18**, 37–121.

Crumpton, M. J. (1974). *In* "The Antigens" (M. Sela, ed.), Vol. 2. Academic Press, New York.

Crumpton, M. J. and Wilkinson, J. M. (1966). *Biochem. J.* **100**, 223–232.

Dreesman, G. R., Sanchez, Y., Ionescu-Matia, I., Sparrow, J. T., Six, H. R., Peterson, D. L., Hollinger, F. B. and Melnick, J. L. (1982). *Nature (London)* **295**, 158–160.

Ellouz, F., Adam, A., Ciorbaru, R. and Lederer, E. (1974). *Biochem. Biophys. Res. Commun.* **59**, 1317–1325.

Freund, J. (1947). *Annu. Rev. Microbiol.* **1**, 291–308.

Fuchs, S., Maoz, A. and Sela, M. (1974). *Israel J. Chem.* **12**, 681–696.

Jackson, D. C., Brown, L. E., White, D. O., Dopheide, T. A. A. and Ward, C. W. (1979). *J. Immunol.* **123**, 2610–2617.

Kotani, S., Watanabe, Y., Kinoshita, F., Shimono, T., Morizaki, L., Shiba, T., Kusimoto, S., Tarumi, Y. and Ikenaka, K. (1975). *Biken. J.* **18**, 105–111.

Langbeheim, H., Arnon, R. and Sela, M. (1976). *Proc. Natl. Acad. Sci. U.S.A.* **73**, 4636–4640.

Lerner, R. A., Green, N., Alexander, H., Liu, F.-T., Sutcliffe, J. G. and Shinnick, T. H. (1981). *Proc. Natl. Acad. Sci. U.S.A.* **78**, 3403–3407.

Liu, U. Y., Tsung, Ch.M. and Fraenkel-Conrat, H. (1967). *J. Mol. Biol.* **24**, 1–14.

Maron, E., Shiozawa, C., Arnon, R. and Sela, M. (1971). *Biochemistry* **10**, 763–771.

Merrifield, B. B. (1965). *Science* **150**, 148–185.

Müller, G., Shapira, M. and Arnon, R. (1982). *Proc. Natl. Acad. Sci. U.S.A.* **79**, 569–573.

Pecht, I., Maron, E., Arnon, R. and Sela, M. (1971). *Eur. J. Biochem.* **19**, 369–371.

Sela, M., Schechter, B., Schechter, I. and Borek, F. (1967). *Cold Spring Harbor Symp. Quant. Biol.* **32**, 537–545.

Teicher, E., Maron, E. and Arnon, R. (1973). *Immunochemistry,* **10**, 265.

Traub, W. and Yonath, A. (1966). *J. Mol. Biol.* **16**, 404–414.

Tsugita, A., Gish, D., Joung, J., Fraenkel-Conrat, H., Knight, C. A. and Stanley, W. M. (1960). *Proc. Natl. Acad. Sci. U.S.A.* **46**, 1463–1469.

Vasquez, C., Granboulan, N. and Franklin, R. M. (1966). *J. Bacteriol.* **92**, 1779–1786.

Weber, K. and Koenigsberg, W. (1975). *In* "RNA-Phages," pp. 51–84. Cold Spring Harbor Laboratory, New York.

Wiley, D. C., Wilson, I. A. and Skehel, J. J. (1981). *Nature (London)* **289**, 366–373.

5

Idiotype Vaccines

F. C. HAY, Y. THANAVALA AND I. M. ROITT

Department of Immunology,
Middlesex Hospital Medical School,
London, England

I. IDIOTYPES

The antigen binding region on the antibody molecule is based on six hypervariable loops, three on the light and three on the heavy chain, which show extraordinary diversity in amino acid sequence (Fig. 1a and b). The area that makes contact with the antigen is called the *paratope*, and even for a single antibody molecule, it is clear that different areas within the hypervariable regions may be used for combining with different antigens. In essence, it only needs sufficient complementarity between the antigen and antibody to generate enough attractive force to enable the secondary conse-

IMMUNE INTERVENTION

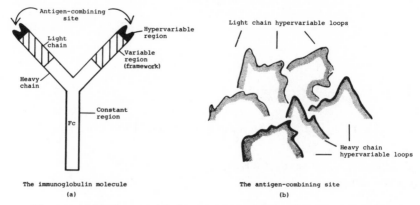

The immunoglobulin molecule
(a)

The antigen-combining site
(b)

Fig. 1.   (a) The immunoglobulin molecule is made up of two heavy and two light chains with hypervariable regions (differing considerably in amino acid sequence from one antibody to another), which form the combining sites for antigen. (b) This combining site may be envisaged as a region of six peaks formed by the hypervariable peptide loops on heavy and light chains with a valley in between them.

quences of antigen binding (e.g., complement fixation, induction of phagocytosis, lymphocyte triggering through receptors) to come into play. This means that a single antibody can combine with a range of antigens in the same way that a single glove can fit many individuals and yet still function as a glove.

If monoclonal antibodies, i.e., a set of structurally identical immunoglobulins produced by a clone of cells all derived from a single progenitor, are used to immunise an animal of another species, antibodies reacting with the constant and variable portions of the monoclonal protein will be formed, and after absorption with pooled normal immunoglobulin, we will be left with antibodies reacting solely with the hypervariable regions. The first studies of this type (Slater *et al.,* 1955) produced absorbed antisera with remarkable specificity for the original monoclonal immunoglobulin showing no cross-reaction with other monoclonals; each antiserum recognizes a number of individual areas or determinants on the hypervariable surface termed *idiotopes,* and the unique collection of idiotopes on each monoclonal immunoglobulin is referred to as an *idiotype.* Just as antigen is defined by antibody, so idiotype is defined by the *anti-idiotypic* reagent, in this case the absorbed antiserum.

The antigen-binding site, or paratope, may or may not be the same as that recognized by anti-idiotype (Fig. 2). In other words, the idiotope(s) may or may not be associated with the same structural region as the paratope in which case we would speak of antigen binding site related or unrelated idiotopes, or if we were hardened professionals, of *paratopic* and *nonparatopic* idiotopes!

In their pioneering studies, Slater *et al.* (1955), Kunkel *et al.* (1963), and Oudin and Michel (1963) independently demonstrated the unique specificity of their anti-idiotypic reagents for the antibodies with which they react, and indeed the very term *idiotype* was employed to convey that uniqueness. However, with a number of systems, it has been shown that different antibodies may share an idiotype or have similar idiotopes as recognized by an anti-idiotype. Idiotypes restricted to a single immunoglobulin are called *private idiotypes* and those common to more than one immunoglobulin, *public* or *cross-reactive* idiotypes (CRI). Advances in our

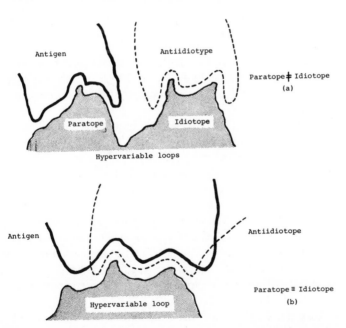

Fig. 2.   The paratope, i.e., that part of the combining site that makes contact with antigen may not be (a) or may be (b) the same as that recognized by the anti-idiotope.

understanding of immunoglobulin genes have revealed that the tremendous diversity of antibodies produced by each individual stems in part from recombination events at the DNA level between various germ line genes and in part from subsequent somatic mutations. The germ line gene products will appear in several different antibodies, presumably giving rise to cross-reactive idiotypes, whereas the rarer structures coded for by random somatic mutations in the germ line genes will be perceived as private idiotypes. Thus CRI tend to be inherited, whereas private idiotypes are not.

II. JERNE'S IDIOTYPE NETWORK HYPOTHESIS

The total number of different hypervariable regions generated by DNA recombination and somatic mutation has been put at around 10^8, although this is by no means a precise figure. If we accept also that each antibody may be capable of combining with several different antigens as discussed, the available repertoire of combining specificities must allow the recognition of virtually every possible molecular shape in the external world. This is one of the major strengths of the lymphocyte immune system because the survival of the species may depend upon the ability to make antibodies to future microbial mutants with surface shapes (determinants) not yet in existence.

Jerne (1974) argued that if the lymphocytes could recognize virtually all possible shapes, they should be able to recognize the hypervariable shapes on the receptors of other lymphocytes. Idiotypes on one lymphocyte would interact with what would be tantamount to the anti-idiotype on another. These mutual idiotypic interactions between lymphocytes would form a vast web or network spreading throughout the lymphocyte repertoire of each individual (Fig. 3). The feasibility of such internal relationships is strongly supported by the ability of monoclonal immunoglobulins and of purified antibodies to raise anti-idiotypes not just in other species, but also in other members of the same species, and most important of all, in syngeneic animals.

Jerne originally envisaged that all lymphocytes were in a state of dynamic equilibrium mediated by these idiotypic interactions. Antigens, merely by disturbing this equilibrium, would provoke an

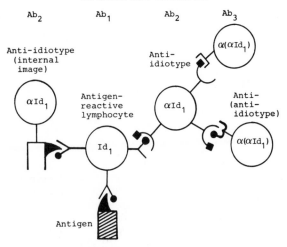

Fig. 3. Elements in an idiotypic network in which the antigen receptors on one lymphocyte recognise an idiotope on the receptors of another (α is used in this and subsequent figures to mean "anti-").

immune response. However, some idiotypes are particularly private, and it is difficult to imagine that there would be sufficiently frequent interactions between very rare idiotypes and their anti-idiotypes to expect any significant contribution to the immune response. On the other hand, public idiotypes are by definition much more common, and there is increasing evidence that they may participate in regulatory immunological processes.

There has been a series of investigations based on the following protocol. The antigen is injected into animal 1 and the antibody produced, Ab_1 (idiotype) is purified and injected into animal 2. Ab_2 (anti-idiotype) so formed is purified and used to immunize animal 3, and so on (Fig. 4). Consistently, it has been found that Ab_2 (anti-Id) recognizes an idiotype (Id) on Ab_1 that is also strongly present in Ab_3. Ab_4 behaves like Ab_2 in seeing the common idiotype on Ab_1 and Ab_3. Nonetheless, although Ab_1 and Ab_3 share idiotypes, only a small fraction of Ab_3 reacts with the original antigen. This is the result one would expect if the idiotype was a CRI (public Id) present on a variety of antibodies (and by implication B-cell receptors) of different specificities. As may be seen in Fig. 4, the anti-Id (Ab_2) when injected into animal 3, would react with all B cells bearing

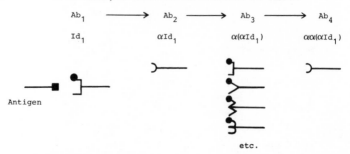

Fig. 4. Ab_1 produced by the antigen is injected into a second animal to produce Ab_2; this in turn is purified and injected into animal 3 and so on. Ab_2 and Ab_4 both react with an idiotype (●) on Ab_1 and Ab_3 but only a fraction of Ab_3 reacts with the original antigen. Paul and Bona (1982) interpret the results in terms of a common idiotype, Id_1, shared by many antibodies other than those reacting with the original antigen but recruited by the injection of anti-Id_1 (Ab_2), which stimulates the range of lymphocytes whose receptors bear the common or cross-reacting idiotype.

the Id and presumably triggers them to produce Id^+ antibodies, only a fraction of which has specificity for the original antigen.

These results suggest that branching of the network at the Ab_2 to Ab_3 stage (cf., Fig. 3) is relatively insignificant. They also indicate why it is that during the course of an immune response, a large number of Id^+ antibodies lacking specificity for antigen may be

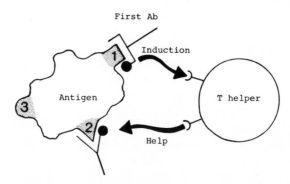

Fig. 5.   The first antibody directed to epitope 1 on the antigen bears a cross-reactive idiotype (●), which stimulates T helpers that recognize the idiotype; the T helpers in turn selectively recruit those lymphocytes with specificity for the other determinants (2 and 3) on the antigen that also bear the cross-reactive idiotype. (Based on the work of Metzger *et al.*, 1981.)

generated (the Oudin and Cazenave paradox, 1971). It is also interesting to note that non-cross-reacting antibodies directed to totally different epitopes on the same antigen may bear the same CRI (Fig. 5) (Cazenave and Oudin, 1973; Cazenave, 1973). One interpretation is that the first clone of antibodies to be formed that bears a dominant CRI generates clonal expansion of helper T cells, which recognize this CRI. Out of all the lymphocytes specific for the other epitopes on the antigen, these T helpers selectively recruit those with CRI positive receptors. It must be noted that this sharing of CRI has not been found in all systems examined (Sakato *et al.*, 1980).

III. PERTURBATION OF THE IMMUNE NETWORK BY ANTI-IDIOTYPE

Administration of anti-idiotype may have many different effects on the immune system depending on which part of the network interacts with the anti-Id. Anti-idiotype may stimulate B cells or helper T cells, thus enhancing the response, or it may act negatively on these cells and mediate suppression. An enhanced response may even be obtained by anti-Id suppression of suppressor cells. The class of antibody, amount administered, and the route of injection all affect the way in which anti-Id can act.

Eichmann (1974) showed that the subclass of an anti-Id determined the outcome of the immune manipulation. Noncomplement fixing guinea pig IgG1 anti-Id (raised to idiotypic determinants on the dominant A5A clone of mouse antibodies to group A streptococcal carbohydrate) when injected into mice selectively enhanced the relevant idiotype, whereas the complement fixing IgG2 fraction of the same antiserum suppressed the idiotype. Similarly, in the (4-hydroxy-3-nitrophenyl)acetyl (NP) system, IgG1 or IgG2a mouse monoclonal anti-Ids were found to, respectively, enhance or suppress the corresponding idiotypes (Reth *et al.*, 1981). However, Sacks *et al.* (1983) have recently reported work from K. Rajewsky showing that IgG2a class-switch mutants of an IgG1 monoclonal anti-Id have identical enhancing properties to the original IgG1 molecule, indicating that regulation associated with isotype may be more complex than at first thought.

In inbred mice the ability to achieve suppression or enhancement is dependent on the amount of anti-Id used, with low doses of the order of 10 ng of monoclonal anti-Id enhancing and high doses around 10 μg suppressing the idiotype in a primary response. The suppressive properties of high doses of both IgG1 and IgG2 in the mouse may be a result of both these subclasses fixing complement in contrast to only IgG2 having this property in guinea pigs.

The route of immunization is also critical; subcutaneous injections of anti-Id promoting delayed hypersensitivity (DTH), but intravenous injections suppressing the response. In contrast, if F(ab')$_2$ fragments of an anti-CRI are used instead of whole molecules, DTH is induced rather than suppressed.

Induction of Antibody by Anti-Id Administration

Injection of an anti-Id can result in (1) selective priming for a dominant idiotype with the resultant subsequent production of idiotypically restricted antibody upon boosting with antigen, or (2) the direct production of specific antibody in the absence of antigen.

1. *Priming*. Minute amounts of guinea pig IgG1 anti-Id injected into mice resulted in the sensitization of both T and B lymphocytes bearing the recurrent A5A idiotype. Limiting dilution experiments have shown that Id$^+$ precursor B cells may be increased from a frequency of 1:2500 to 1:200 by preimmunization with IgG1 anti-Id (Eichmann *et al.*, 1977). Thus, in the absence of antigen, a more than 10-fold increase in the Id bearing B-cell population occurred. An interesting aspect of these studies was that the numbers of Id$^+$ nonantigen binding clones was enhanced in parallel with antigen binding Id$^+$ clones in both antigen and anti-Id treated animals, showing that B-cell populations defined entirely by idiotype undergo quantitative changes, even if only a certain portion of them interact with antigen in a detectable manner. In the A5A system both the antigen binding and nonantigen binding, but Id$^+$ immunoglobulins share the same V_H segment gene. Presumably the CRI is situated in this region and is stimulated independently of antigen binding properties dependent on the D and J_H segments of the variable region (Fig. 6) (Margolies *et al.*, 1983).

Adoptive transfer and *in vitro* culture experiments have demonstrated that anti-Id can sensitize T cells bearing the relevant Id to

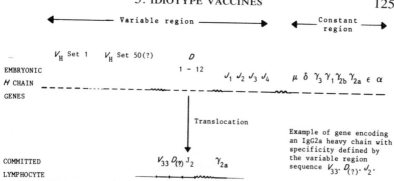

Fig. 6.   Genes coding for κ and heavy chain peptides in the mouse. The genetic basis for the highly variable D segment in the heavy chain which lies between the V and J segments is uncertain.

provide help for the production of Id bearing immunoglobulins (Eichmann and Rajewsky, 1975; Cosenza et al., 1977). When spleen cells from A/J mice presensitized with either streptococcal A antigen or guinea pig IgG1 anti-Id (raised against the A5A idiotype) were cultured with strep A conjugated to the trinitrophenyl (TNP) hapten, TNP-specific plaque-forming cells were generated in almost equal numbers in each group, indicating that T cell help had been successfully generated to the strep A carrier. Anti-Id generation of Id-specific helper T cells is now well documented (Gleason et al., 1981; Sachs et al., 1981; Miller et al., 1981, 1982), but it is also possible to induce help for an idiotype that the animal would not normally produce in response to antigen. Immunization of BALB/c and B10/D2 mice with staphylococcal nuclease antigen leads to the production of antinuclease antibody bearing different idiotypes in the two strains. It was possible, however, to induce the production of BALB/c Id-bearing nonantigen binding molecules in both strains by treating with pig anti-BALB/c Id. This same treatment was able to produce helper T cells bearing the BALB/c Id in both strains. These helper T cells were able to provide antigen-specific help even in the B10/D2 mice despite the inability of the Id⁺ immunoglobulins in that strain to bind antigen specifically (cf. Fig. 7b).

Not only can administration of anti-Id lead directly to the stimulation of Id-bearing helper T cells, but an enhanced Id response may also be due to the elimination of T-suppressor cells specific for the idiotype (Bona *et al.*, 1979). Production of a specific Id can also be driven by helper T cells bearing anti-Id, which can interact directly with B cells bearing the idiotype (Cerny and Caulfield, 1981).

2. *Antibody production.* Although frequently anti-Id treatment leads solely to priming (Fig. 7a), in some situations antibody may be produced. Take, for example, the T15 Id, which represents the dominant CRI in the antibody response to pneumococcal antigens containing multiple phosphoryl choline (PC) residues in many strains of mice. *In vitro* studies have shown that in the absence of antigen an anti-PC T15$^+$ plaque-forming cell response was induced with anti-Id that was comparable to that generated by the antigen itself (Cammisuli and Cosenza, 1980) (Fig. 7b). *In vivo,* the production of specific antibody following anti-Id has been shown to occur both within and across a species barrier. Trenkner and Riblett (1975) induced PC antibody both *in vivo* and *in vitro* in mice given rabbit anti-Id. *In vivo* the response generated was 20% of that obtained by immunising with antigen. When antigen and anti-Id were given together the response was not merely additive but was twice the expected sum. Anti-Id has also been used to generate antibody to histocompatibility antigens. Anti-Id was raised in rabbits and guinea pigs to mouse monoclonal antibodies to H-2K^k. Mice treated with these anti-Id reagents, in the absence of antigen, consistently produced large amounts of Id. In some of the mice, a proportion of the response included Id$^+$ antibody, which bound to H-2K^k antigens (Bluestone *et al.*, 1981).

Syngeneic systems may also sometimes produce antibody *in vivo*. BALB/c mice given BALB/c anti-Id in a TNP system produced a very strong Id$^+$ response compared with mice injected with antigen, and a small proportion of this was specific anti-TNP antibody (Bernabe *et al.*, 1981). Rabbits may also be induced to form antibody in the absence of antigen. Couraud *et al.* (1983) raised anti-Id to rabbit alprenolol antibody. These rabbits then produced auto-anti-anti-Id (Ab$_3$) some of which bound the original antigen.

Not only is there evidence that anti-Id treatment induces specific antibody, but also this antibody can be biologically useful. Sacks *et al.* (1982) immunised mice with polyclonal mouse anti-Id, raised

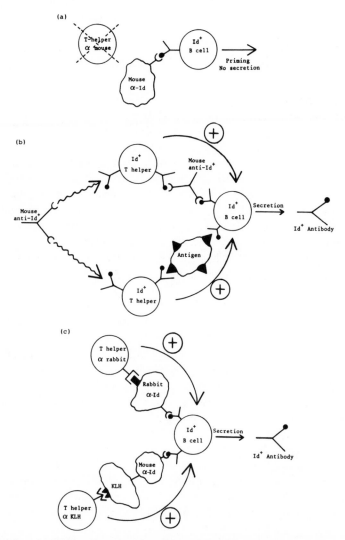

Fig. 7.   (a) Id⁺ B cells primed by mouse anti-Id but in the absence of T cell help, no antibody is secreted; (b) Id⁺ B cells stimulated by Id⁺ T helpers operating through anti-idiotype or antigen with repeating epitopes; (c) Id⁺ B cells stimulated (⊕) by T helpers directed to heterologous carrier.

against mouse monoclonal antitrypanosomal antibody, and they were able to protect these mice from infection with the homologous African trypanosomes.

Why then does anti-Id sometimes induce antibody but on other occasions only prime the response? One of the key requirements appears to be the presence of T-cell help. In Trenkner and Riblett's (1975) experiments on induction of antibody in mice with rabbit anti-Id, no induction was obtained if the mouse T cells were tolerised to normal rabbit IgG, but the response was restored if T cells educated against rabbit IgG were added to the tolerised cultures (Fig. 7c). Similarly Rajewsky's group have previously shown that mouse monoclonal anti-Ids given to mice were able to sensitise but did not provoke antibody production. Now, however, by chemically cross-linking the anti-Id to keyhole limpet haemocyanin and so providing an effective carrier molecule they converted the anti-Ids to potent immunogens (Takemori et al., 1982) (Fig. 7c).

Use of these anti-CRI has shown that effective antigen binding Id$^+$ antibody molecules may be induced within the same strain, but sometimes when other strains are immunized, Id$^+$ molecules are induced that do not bind antigen. The control of the Id repertoire appears to be linked to the IgH locus and reflects V gene polymorphisms, with most CRI being associated with the V segment. Because of differences in association of various D and J segments with a particular V segment, antigen binding may be dissociated from the CRI, the CRI probably being on a part of the combining site outside the antigen binding site (Fig. 2a). If an Id could be located within the antigen binding site of an antibody, this could lead to the production of an anti-Id, which would fit into the combining site (Fig. 2b). Given a binding site Id, which closely fitted an epitope on the antigen, then an anti-Id, which was accurately complementary in shape to the Id, would be similar to the three-dimensional shape of the antigen and would represent the "internal image" of that particular antigenic epitope in the immune system.

IV. EVIDENCE FOR "INTERNAL IMAGE"

Considerable evidence has now been obtained supporting the original view of Jerne (1974) and Lindenmann (1973) that anti-Id may take on the shape of part of the antigen molecule and give rise to an internal image of the antigen. Several situations where internal image has been demonstrated have involved anti-Ids mimicking hormones, which has allowed use of the tissue hormone receptors as a detection system for the anti-Id. These systems are extremely sensitive and capable of revealing small amounts of anti-Id beyond the limits of detection of conventional radioimmunoassays. In one of the first demonstrations of internal image, rabbit anti-Id was prepared against rat antibodies to retinol binding protein (RBP) or insulin (Sege and Peterson, 1978). The RBP anti-Id was able to bind to rat intestinal epithelial cells and prevent the uptake of retinol from RBP, whereas the insulin anti-Ids could inhibit the binding of insulin to rat epididymal fat cells, although mg amounts of IgG were needed in each system. Despite these positive results, the IgG fractions did not contain measurable amounts of insulin or RBP determinants, as determined by radioimmunoassay, indicating that there were either very few immunoglobulin molecules resembling the antigens or that the anti-Ids were only a poor representation of the antigens. Shechter *et al.* (1982) have also found anti-Id resembling insulin although in their experiments the animals were immunised with insulin itself. Both antiinsulin and its corresponding anti-Id were produced, the latter being detected by demonstrating its insulin-like activity on the metabolism of fat cells.

Internal image has been shown with anti-Id antibodies capable of binding to β-adrenergic receptors. Rabbits were immunized with alprenolol (a β-adrenergic antagonist) and anti-Id was prepared against this Ab1. The anti-Id was found to agglutinate turkey red blood cells (which have β-adrenergic receptors) but not human or sheep red blood cells, which lack the receptors. The binding of dihydroalprenolol could be inhibited by the anti-Id, and the binding to receptor was not simply passive as basal adenylate cyclase activity was stimulated (Schreiber *et al.*, 1980). Independently, Homcy *et al.* (1982) have produced anti-Id, which also bound the β-adrenergic receptor, but behaved differently in inhibition studies.

Another approach to recognising internal image anti-Id is to determine whether the anti-Id is bound by antibodies to the original antigen, raised in other species. It is unlikely that these other species will produce antibody with the same idiotype as the original antibody and are only likely to bind the anti-Id if it bears determinants resembling the antigen. Urbain *et al.* (1980) found one remarkable anti-Id, produced in a rabbit, against antibody to tobacco mosaic virus (TMV). This anti-Id bound antibodies to TMV from every rabbit examined and also antibody from mice, horses, goats and chickens immunized with TMV. Most importantly, the anti-Id induced the formation of anti-TMV when injected into mice. This anti-Id must constitute one of the most perfect examples of internal image so far encountered, but it was only one out of several hundred rabbits that produced this specificity. Marasco and Becker (1982) followed a similar line of reasoning using the chemoattractant formyl peptide, fMet-Leu-Phe as antigen. Rabbit antibodies were prepared to fMet-Leu-Phe and given to mice, guinea pigs, and a goat. Some of the goat anti-Id bound to nearly every rabbit and rat anti-fMet-Leu-Phe antibody examined. Further, $F(ab')_2$ of the anti-Id bound to the receptors for fMet-Leu-Phe on polymorphonuclear leucocytes.

Recently, Cazenave et al. (1983) have shown that the recurrent idiotypes they previously demonstrated in the rabbit allotype system may be accounted for by the presence of internal images in their anti-idiotype preparation. These internal images of rabbit b6 allotype could be induced in both rabbits and mice.

How common are internal image-bearing lymphocytes? Looking at the generation first of Id and then of anti-Id in Fig. 8, it is clear from our knowledge of antibody responses that only a small fraction of the Id molecules will be accurately complementary to the antigen and in the next stage, we would expect only a small fraction of these particular Ids to induce the formation of anti-Ids with sufficient high fidelity complementarity to resemble the original antigen. Tasiaux et al. (1978) counted peripheral blood lymphocytes producing auto-anti-Id capable of binding fluorescent anti-TMV from the same rabbit and found from 0.1 to 0.5% of lymphocytes positive. Jackson et al. (1981) found far higher numbers of anti-Id bearing cells when they examined lymphocytes from the spleen. Following prolonged immunisation of rabbits with human serum albumin or human lactoferrin, they removed the spleens and looked for cells producing auto-anti-Id. These were detected with fluorescent conjugates of the $F(ab')_2$ fraction prepared from the antibody that each rabbit had produced at an early stage. From 0.7 to 44% of cells bound the antibody in different rabbits. Further, they were able to take anti-bovine serum albumin (BSA) from other

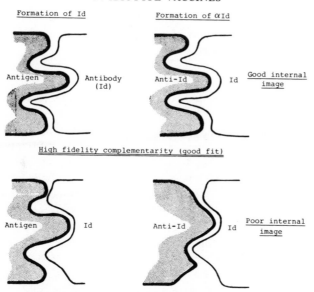

Fig. 8.   The accuracy with which the idiotypic antibody fits the antigen and the subsequent accuracy of interaction with the anti-idiotype determines how similar the shape of the anti-idiotype is to the antigen, i.e., how accurate an "internal image" it is.

species such as chickens and show that this was bound by 2 to 40% of spleen plasma cells from rabbits immunized with BSA; assuming that the findings were not complicated by the presence of residual antigen, they would suggest that an internal image was being produced. Recently, we have been able to demonstrate mouse spleen cells bearing the internal image of human chorionic gonadotropin (hCG) in mice immunised with hCG. These were revealed with fluorescent rabbit anti-hCG but were present in very low numbers.

It is perhaps pertinent to note that so far no demonstrations of internal image have been made with monoclonal antibodies. All the examples so far have followed immunisation with polyclonal antibody populations or with antigen. It may well be that in heterogeneous antisera consisting of a whole spectrum of antibody molecules, the predominant feature may be the average of the paratopic (antigen binding) sites rather than individual idiotopes, and correspondingly the common feature in a polyclonal anti-Id serum could be the internal image of the antigen.

V. STRATEGY FOR VACCINE BASED ON ANTI-Id

Stimulation of lymphocyte receptors with either antigen or internal image anti-Id should turn on similar populations of lymphocytes bearing various idiotypes. If a noninternal image anti-Id is used, this will stimulate only the subpopulation of cells with that idiotype. This set will not necessarily be the same as the antigen binding set and is very likely to include a majority of cells that have the idiotype but do not bind antigen. This may not present a real problem as Sacks and Sher (1983) have recently shown that even though their stimulated, antigen-specific idiotype was only formed in small amounts, this was biologically active enough to protect mice against trypanosome infection. Operationally, idiotype heterogeneity can be difficult as idiotype diversity is generally greater than amino acid sequence diversity. Pairs of myeloma proteins binding dextran have been shown to differ by more idiotypes than amino acid substitutions (reviewed by Rudikoff, 1983). Conversely, examination of antibodies produced by mutant cells has revealed that single amino acid changes may destroy antigen binding completely without necessarily altering the binding of anti-Id (Rudikoff et al., 1982).

In certain situations, the number of genes contributing to an antibody response is very small, leading to restricted heterogeneity. In the phosphocholine system, the heavy chains of myeloma proteins binding phosphocholine are similar in sequence and are all members of the same subgroup in all inbred mouse strains tested. Those differences that do occur in heavy chains from different strains are principally in the D segment, with the first two hypervariable regions being very similar and often identical. The differences in D segments appear to make little difference to the antigen binding properties. Clearly, where there is this restricted heterogeneity, anti-Ids directed against idiotopes on the first two hypervariable regions are going to induce the production of the relevant antibody in all strains. Perhaps, this germline presence of certain antibody *V* genes in all mice reflects the importance of these antibodies for survival.

More frequently anti-Ids are raised to variable region determinants, which are restricted in that they are only associated with particular antigen binding specificities in mice possessing the same heavy chain constant region allotypes, as seen with antibodies to the NP hapten (Takemori *et al.*, 1982) or to trypanosomes (Sacks and Sher, 1983). This may reflect polymorphism of the structural genes encoding the heavy chain phenotypes. Primi *et al.* (1981) have, however, proposed that allotype linkage of Id expression may be due to regulatory cells that recognize Id only in conjunction with certain allotypes. If different V-region polymorphisms are generally found in separate strains, this will make anti-Id manipulations difficult in outbred populations.

We are considering two possible pathways for tackling this problem. One involves manipulating Id-specific T cells. We have already mentioned the ability of heterologous anti-BALB/c Id to prime nuclease-specific splenic helper T cells in a strain which does not normally produce antibodies with the BALB/c Id (Miller *et al.*, 1982). This could be especially helpful where T cells provide the effector arm against infectious organisms (Playfair *et al.*, 1977). In contrast, it must be remembered that anti-A5A Id failed to sensitize helper T cells in those strains not normally producing A5A Id in their response to Group A Streptococci (Black *et al.*, 1976; Eichmann and Rajewsky, 1975), indicating that different conditions may apply to each antigen.

The second approach is to use anti-Ids which mimic the antigen. To test the potential of internal image anti-Ids as vaccines of the future necessitates their production on a large scale. The recent advances in the development of monoclonal antibodies from hybridomas make it possible to obtain large quantities of anti-Id. Obviously, it would be ideal to use monoclonal antibodies at each stage. Antigen, not necessarily highly purified, could be used to produce monoclonal antibody (idiotype), and this in turn could be used to raise monoclonal anti-Id. Internal image anti-Id would be identified by testing for its antigen-like behaviour, where the antigen has biological activity or by examining its binding to antisera, prepared in other species, to the initial antigen. The relative infrequency with which internal image anti-Ids have been found may make it necessary to enrich the lymphocyte population for this before fusion by using heterologous antibodies to the original antigen for coating plates to "pan" cells or for labelling cells before fractionation in a fluorescence activated cell sorter (FACS). Selective expansion of the total anti-Id pool may be helpful and could be achieved by treatment *in vivo* or *in vitro* with Id coupled to a polyclonal activator such as lipopolysaccharide.

The possibility remains, however, that monoclonal idiotype may not be the best reagent for raising internal image anti-Id. When a monoclonal antibody is injected into a mouse all the variable portions of the variable region are potentially immunogenic and antibodies will be raised to every one of idiotypic determinants presented on the antibody molecule. Internal image Ids binding intimately with the paratopic site will be only a small proportion of these. In fact, if the paratope is formed by a cleft this may be the least immunogenic portion of the molecule. If instead, a polyclonal antiserum is used, preferably from a pool of outbred animals or even different species, each individual idiotope will only form a very small proportion of the total, but the common feature shared by all the various antibodies will be the paratopic site as they all bind to the same antigenic determinant. Thus the major stimulation will be directed towards lymphocytes bearing internal image that can bind any or all of these antibodies.

VI. ADVANTAGES OF MONOCLONAL INTERNAL IMAGE ANTI-Id VACCINES

There are several circumstances in which the use of conventional vaccination presents certain problems and in these cases internal image anti-Id vaccine may prove useful.

A. Difficulty in Obtaining Adequate Amounts of Antigen

The lack of adequate amounts of antigen has been one of the key factors in our present failure to produce appropriate vaccines for a wide range of diseases, such as malaria, trypanosomiasis, filariasis, leprosy, and leishmaniasis. In all these cases, the organisms are difficult to grow in large numbers, whereas in certain infectious diseases, for example hepatitis B, it is not even possible to culture the virus *in vitro*.

In all these situations monoclonal anti-Id which would serve as surrogate antigens could be easily produced on a large scale.

B. Defective Configuration of Antigens by Gene Cloning or Peptide Synthesis

Apart from the problems associated with the efficient large-scale production of proteins by genetic engineering, the products so obtained may not be of value for use as a vaccine if they require glycosylation or the presence of lipid or the nucleic acid core (as in entero-viruses) to attain the configuration of the native antigen.

Similarly, a synthetic peptide may not fold correctly to provide the required three-dimensional structure of the original antigen and may therefore prove to be a weaker antigen. Although no formal proof exists, suggestive evidence for this argument comes from the work performed with the synthetic C-terminal peptide of β-hCG, which is used by the WHO programme for the control of fertility, which provoked antibodies with only low affinity for the parent hCG molecule. Internal image set anti-Id would have the correct conformation and thus in this context be a more potent antigen.

There are, however, instances where the products of gene cloning or synthetic vaccines could prove very successful as in the recent studies with hepatitis B virus surface antigen (Smith *et al.*, 1983).

C. Disadvantages Associated with Conventional Vaccines Using Microorganisms

In the early days of killed polio vaccine, it was found that live virus was present in some batches of vaccine that produced paralytic polio myelitis in some children illustrating the inherent hazards associated with the use of putatively killed vaccines and stresses the need for very stringent measures to ensure that such vaccines are safe and stable. There is the risk also with attenuated strains of reversion to the virulent form. Monoclonal antibodies are not infectious agents, and their use as vaccines would circumvent the dangers associated with both killed and attenuated organisms.

D. Immunity to a Single Determinant Only Is Required

Sometimes determinants of a microbial antigen not needed for immune protection, or complexes of the organisms with body components may provoke autoantibodies that could be damaging. It is thought that streptococcal strains that cause rheumatic fever and *T. cruzi,* the causative agent of Chagas' disease, both cross-react with heart tissue. Thus, vaccines directed to the entire organisms might also produce reactivity against normal body components, and it would therefore be an advantage to immunize only against selected protective antigenic determinants.

Infection with strain 1 dengue virus protects against the homologous strain, but subsequent infection with the related strain 2 leads to severe haemorrhagic disease as a paradoxical result of cross-reactive antibodies produced by the strain 1 virus. A vaccine that produced immunity to only strain-specific determinants and not to cross-reacting epitopes would be beneficial because there would be less chance of haemorrhagic disease in individuals responding poorly to any given strain. Similarly, it might also be important to immunise against single determinants on respiratory syncytial virus and measles virus if it proved to be the case that haemorrhagic disease due to reinfection during the waning of immunity produced by killed vaccines was a consequence of sensitisation to nonprotective determinants. With new strains of infuenza virus produced by antigenic drift, it could be an advantage to immunise against the new determinants if the whole virus tends to drive the immune response to produce antibodies towards an earlier infective strain (''original antigenic sin''). Monoclonal anti-Ids again have an advantage in that they provide a means of immunising against single antigenic determinants.

Accepting that anti-Id vaccines have significant advantages, how practical is this approach to vaccine development? In outbred populations, anti-Ids that are not antigen combining site-related are unlikely to be successful in stimulating B cells for specific antibody production. As discussed, however, they may be capable of T-cell priming, which would be of value where defence is largely dependent on T effectors directed against particular epitopes, and might also permit better co-operative antibody responses on natural infection with the organism. It is our view that the monoclonal internal image anti-Id represents a highly desirable goal as this should stimulate specific antibody regardless of *V*-gene polymorphisms. The production of these reagents will entail screening many anti-Ids, but it may prove essential to enhance their selection by techniques of specific enrichment of appropriate B cells, as suggested earlier.

ACKNOWLEDGEMENTS

We are grateful to the Medical Research Council for supporting our research on idiotype vaccines, and to Miss C. Meats for her invaluable secretarial assistance in the preparation of the manuscript and her contribution to the artwork.

REFERENCES

Bernabe, R. R., Coutinho, A., Martinez, A. C. and Cazenave, P. A. (1981). *J. Exp. Med.* **154**, 552.

Black, S. J., Hammerling, G. J., Berek, C., Rajewsky, K. and Eichmann, K. (1976). *J. Exp. Med.* **143**, 846.

Bluestone, J. A., Sharrow, S. O., Epstein, S. L., Ozato, K. and Sachs, D. H. (1981). *Nature (London)* **291**, 233.

Bona, C., Hooghe, R., Cazenave, P. A., Leguèrn, C. and Paul, W. E. (1979). *J. Exp. Med.* **149**, 815.

Cammisuli, S. and Cosenza, H. (1980). *Eur. J. Immunol.* **10**, 299.

Cazenave, P. A. (1973). *FEBS Lett.* **31**, 348.

Cazenave, P. A. and Oudin, J. (1973). *C. R. Acad. Sci. Paris* **276**, 243.

Cazenave, P. A., Roland, J. and Petit-Koskas, E. (1983). *Ann. Immunol. (Inst.Pasteur)* **134D**, 7.

Cerny, J. and Caulfield, M. J. (1981). *J. Immunol.* **126**, 2262.

Cosenza, H., Julius, M. H. and Augustin, A. A. (1977). *Immunol. Rev.* **34**, 3.

Couraud, P. O., Lu, B. Z. and Strosberg, A. D. (1983). *J. Exp. Med.* **157**, 1369.

Eichmann, K. (1974). *Eur. J. Immunol.* **4**, 296.

Eichmann, K. and Rajewsky, K. (1975). *Eur. J. Immunol.* **5**, 661.

Eichmann, K., Coutinho, A. and Melchers, F. (1977). *J. Exp. Med.* **146**, 1436.

Gleason, K., Pierce, S. and Kohler, H. (1981). *J. Exp. Med.* **153**, 924.

Homcy, C. J., Rockson, S. G. and Haber, E. (1982). *J. Clin. Invest.* **69**, 1147.

Jackson, S., Kulhavy, R. and Mestecky, J. (1981). *Scand. J. Immunol.* **14**, 31.

Jerne, N. K. (1974). *Ann. Immunol. (Inst.Pasteur)* **125c**, 373.

Kunkel, H. G., Mannik, M. and Williams, R. C. (1963). *Science* **140**, 1218.

Lindenmann, J. (1973). *Ann. Immunol. (Inst.Pasteur)* **124c**, 171.

Marasco, W. A. and Becker, E. L. (1982). *J. Immunol.* **128**, 963.

Margolies, M. N., Wysocki, L. J. and Sato, V. L. (1983). *J. Immunol.* **130**, 515.

Metzger, D. W., Furman, A., Miller, A. and Sercarz, E. E. (1981). *J. Exp. Med.* **154**, 701.

Miller, G. G., Nadler, P. I., Asano, Y., Hodes, R. J. and Sachs, D. H. (1981). *J. Exp. Med.* **154**, 24.

Miller, G. G., Nadler, P. I., Hodes, R. J. and Sachs, D. H. (1982). *J. Exp. Med.* **155**, 190.

Oudin, J. and Cazenave, P. A. (1971). *Proc. Natl. Acad. Sci. U.S.A.* **68**, 2616.

Oudin, J. and Michel, M. (1963). *C. R. Acad. Sci.* **257**, 805.

Paul, W. E., and Bona, C. (1982). *Immunol. Today* **3**, 230–234.

Playfair, J. H. L., de Souza, J. B. a.d Cottrell, B. J. (1977). *Immunology* **32**, 681.

Primi, D., Juy, D. and Cazenave, P. A. (1981). *Eur. J. Immunol.* **11**, 393.

Reth, M., Kelsoe, G. and Rajewsky, K. (1981). *Nature (London)* **290**, 257.

Rudikoff, S. (1983). *In* "Contemporary Topics in Molecular Immunology" (F. P. Inman and T. J. Kindt, eds.), Vol. 9, p. 169. Plenum, New York.

Rudikoff, S., Giusti, A., Cook, W. D. and Scharff, M. D. (1982). *Proc. Natl. Acad. Sci.* **79**, 1979.

Sachs, D. H., El-Gamil, M. and Miller, G. (1981). *Eur. J. Immunol.* **11**, 509.

Sacks, D. L. and Sher, A. (1983). *J. Immunol.* **131**, 1511.

Sacks, D. L., Esser, K. M. and Sher, A. (1982). *J. Exp. Med.* **155**, 1108.

Sacks, D. L., Kelsoe, G. H. and Sachs, D. H. (1983). *Springer Sem. Immunopathol.* **6**(1), 79.

Sakato, N., Fujio, H. and Amano, T. (1980). *J. Immunol.* **124**, 1866.

Schreiber, A. B., Couraud, P. O., Andre, C., Vray, B. and Strosberg, A. D. (1980). *Proc. Natl. Acad. Sci. U.S.A.,* **77**, 7385.

Sege, K. and Peterson, P. A. (1978). *Proc. Natl. Acad. Sci. U.S.A.* **75**, 2443.

Shechter, Y., Maron, R., Elias, D. and Cohen, I. R. (1982). *Science* **216**, 542.

Slater, R. J., Ward, S. M. and Kunkel, H. G. (1955). *J. Exp. Med.* **101**, 85.

Smith, G. L., Mackott, M. and Moss, B. (1983). *Nature (London)* **302**, 490.

Takemori, T., Tesch, H., Reth, M. and Rajewsky, K. (1982). *Eur. J. Immunol.* **12**, 1040.

Tasiaux, N., Leuwenkroon, R., Bruyns, C. and Urbain, J. (1978). *Eur. J. Immunol.* **8**, 464.

Trenkner, E. and Riblet, R. (1975). *J. Exp. Med.* **142**, 1121.

Urbain, J., Cazenave, P. A., Wikler, M., Franssen, J. D., Mariame, B. and Leo, O. (1980). *Prog. Immunol.* **IV**, 81.

Index